GREAT BHĀRATA

Founded in 2020, and headquartered in Gainesville, Florida, USA, HDG Global Publications is a non-profit, independent publisher committed to publishing classic spiritual literature, in print and audio formats, that inspire the reader's spiritual evolution.

Based on the ancient Sanskrit literature of South Asia, and adapted for contemporary audiences both lay and academic, our publications make advanced concepts comprehensible and enjoyable.

GREAT BHĀRATA

THE INVASION BEGINS

VOLUME ONE

HOWARD RESNICK, PhD

MANDALA

SAN RAFAEL LOS ANGELES LONDON

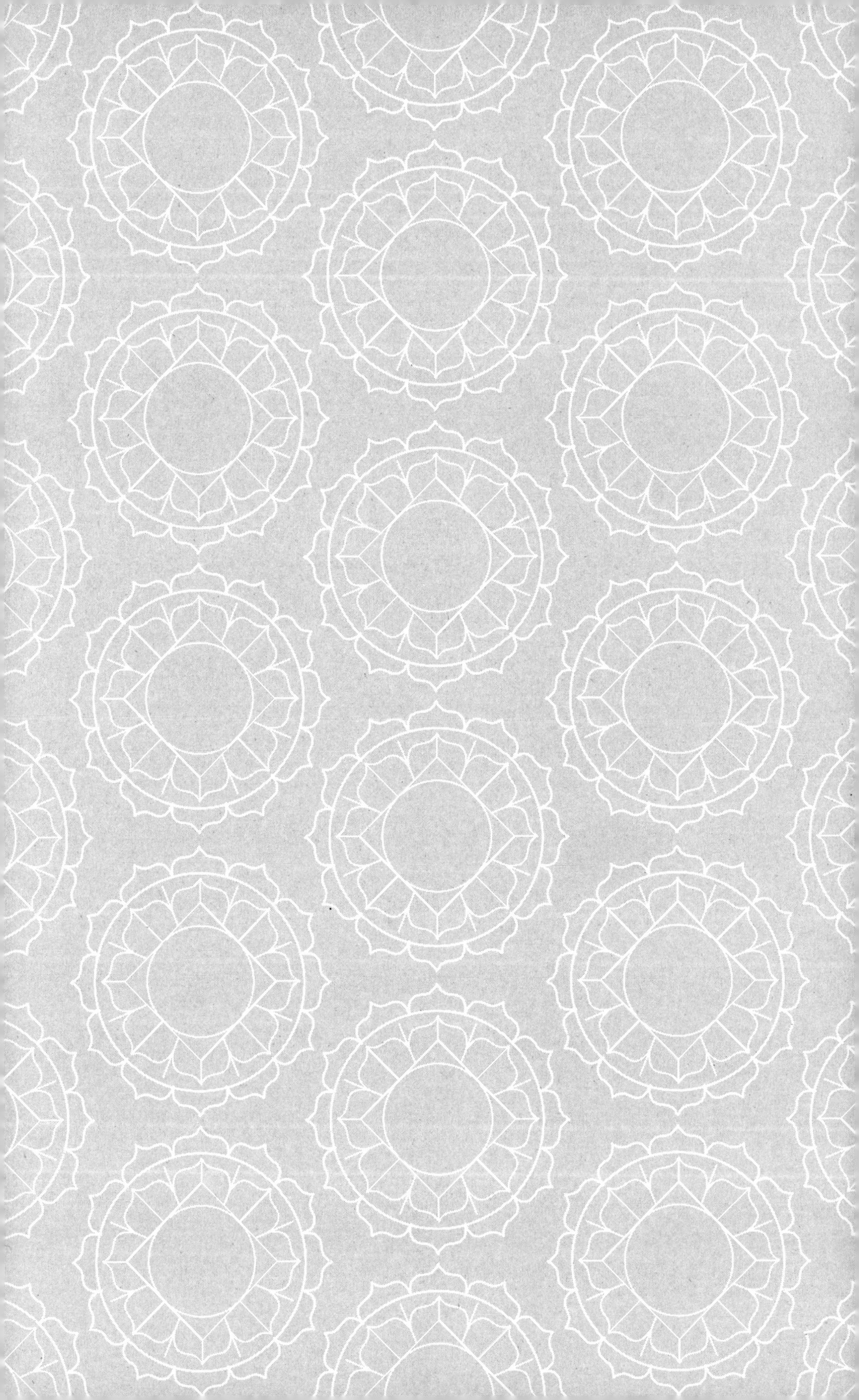

PREFACE

Imagine a global catastrophe. Choose your scenario — nuclear Armageddon, climate cataclysm, or perhaps the second coming of a huge asteroid, like the one that devastated Earth 66 million years ago, abolishing dinosaurs and reinventing our planet.

In our imaginary scenario, miraculously, humanity survives but cannot regenerate our lost civilization in its technically advanced form. Before our scientific and industrial revolutions, humans lived for many thousands of years on this planet in a comparatively simple, basic state. Now, once again, thousands of years pass, but another scientific revolution does not occur.

In that distant future, some of our own books survive. These texts describe the high-tech wonders, the medical miracles, of our present age. But in the distant future, humans living a rudimentary life have no analogues to our technology. So, they do not believe our books and their claims — that one just points and clicks and hills explode, rockets roar into space. One moves a cursor and the blind can see, the lame can walk. For the simple future people who cannot recover or reinvent our world, a true description of our world is mere primitive mythology.

Ancient Sanskrit texts teach that something very much like this has already happened. Many thousands of years ago, a wonderfully advanced subtle science, surviving today only in its most surface remnant as physical yoga, produced a celestial civilization on our planet. Interplanetary intercourse flourished. But a catastrophic world war drained Earth's spirit and resources. Time itself, in a cosmic form unknown to us today, consumed human virtues that sustained exalted human culture.

Long ago, the *Mahā-bhārata* and the *Bhāgavatam,* casting their gaze into the future, asserted that it is we today, with all our proud technology, who are the fallen future people. It is the ancients who built a truly advanced, but now lost, civilization. Yet these same primordial texts assure that hope exists, for they bequeathed to us histories of their fabulous world. These texts also assert that we can recover the higher consciousness of their long-lost civilization, if we can but hear their voices.

Yet because we have no experience of such an advanced world, we tend to reject their accounts and assurances as mere myth — fables and fantasies. Those ancients would tell us that their stories are true and real. But as millennia passed, history decayed into legend, legend sank into myth.

We now embark on a literary voyage that I hope will restore our vision of glorious ancestors and a more enlightened world. While we cannot expect to reconstitute that world in all its powers, we can and should endeavor to reclaim the deepest wisdom that great souls, with great compassion, gave to us in the form of sacred texts.

But how can we be sure that such a world ever existed? I address that natural doubt in the Introduction. Wise people the world over see our desperate need to restore peace and wisdom to a troubled world. Hoping to do my part, I wrote this book. Through its pages, may a forgotten world be recalled to our collective memory. That world, described in *Great Bhārata*, can be our shining guide.

INTRODUCTION

The words *Great Bhārata* translate the Sanskrit *Mahā-bhārata*, the title of an ancient and extraordinary text that claims to tell the immemorial history of South Asia, of the Earth, and indeed of our universe. One of the world's largest books, the *Mahā-bhārata* is three times the size of the Old and New Testament combined, and seven times the combined *Iliad* and *Odyssey*. Its myriad Sanskrit verses have greatly influenced South Asia and beyond for thousands of years.

The *Mahā-bhārata* is often said to focus on an earthly dynastic struggle between two royal families. This depiction is true, but incomplete. In fact, the text weaves its chronicle on three distinct but interlaced levels — earthly, cosmic, and spiritual.

1. Earthly. The text does describe a dynastic struggle between the Kurus and Pāṇḍavas, two powerful royal families.

2. Cosmic. In that royal fight, Earth is merely a proxy battleground for a conflict of cosmic proportions, a true war of the worlds.

3. Spiritual. As the *Bhagavad-gītā* explains in the *Mahā-bhārata*'s Book Six, chapters 23-40, the earthly and cosmic events produced profound spiritual consequences for those involved, and for us today.

The word *Bhārata* derives from *Bharata*, a king so celebrated that the land he ruled became known as *Bhārata, the land of Bharata*. In its native languages, India still bears the name Bhārata.

Naturally, political boundaries have shifted since ancient times. In its original sense, *Bhārata* referred to South Asia and some areas beyond, and to a magnificent civilization that flourished in these and other regions of the world.

Who composed the *Mahā-bhārata* and when? Does it describe real historical events, or mere mythology? What does it ultimately teach?

For centuries, two distinct communities have given very different answers to these questions. One approach, which I will call *secular* scholarship, has grown over the last several centuries, chiefly among Western, and Western-trained, scholars.

The other, and far older, approach emerges from within the ancient Sanskrit culture itself. I will call this method *devotional* scholarship. It sees the text as sacred, historical, and revelatory.

Let us keep in mind that neither secular nor devotional scholarship on the *Mahā-bhārata* is uniform or monolithic within their respective communities. Both groups have always engaged in vigorous *internal* debates.

There are also significant points of agreement between secular and devotional scholars, such as the belief that the Sanskrit text of the *Mahā-bhārata* available to us today in various regional recensions is not a pristine, original text. I will speak more about that later.

Further, these two types of scholarship — secular and devotional — do not exhaust all the historical approaches to understanding the *Mahā-bhārata*. Some scholars simply strive to *describe* secular and devotional claims in the most neutral way possible, rather than giving critical, non-literal interpretations, or making ultimate *metaphysical* claims.

Yet, despite these three factors — a) internal debates among both secular and devotional scholars; b) important agreements between these two groups; and c) attempts to maintain interpretive neutrality, it is still most practical and realistic here to focus on the two primary forms of *Mahā-bhārata* scholarship — secular and devotional, for these are by far the two most influential approaches. They reveal the competing metaphysics of the spiritual and secular approach to the text, and perhaps to life itself.

It is important to note that here and throughout this Introduction, I use the term *metaphysics* (or its cognate *metaphysical*) as applied to the teachings of Aristotle in his treatise of that name.[1] "Aristotle says that 'everyone takes what is called *wisdom* (sophia) to be concerned with the primary causes (aitia) and the starting-points…(981b28), and it is these causes and principles that he proposes

1 Aristotle himself did not use the term. A few centuries later, the name *Metaphysics* was given to his treatise. Thus, the topics in that work came to be known as metaphysics.

to study..." Similarly, Aristotle claims that he will discuss "a science that studies things...that are eternal, not subject to change, and independent of matter. Aristotle states that such a science is theology,... the "first" and "highest" science."[2]

For over 1500 years, Western philosophy took the topics discussed in Aristotle's *Metaphysics* to be the proper subjects of metaphysics, as they continue to be for some contemporary philosophers. Since Aristotle, the *first cause* or *unmoved mover* has often been identified with God in some form.

This Aristotelian notion of the first and most important area of philosophy closely matches the teachings of the *Bhagavad-gītā*,[3] and we must pay close attention to Kṛṣṇa's treatise if we are to grasp the significance of the *Mahā-bhārata*, the *Bhāgavatam*, and many other ancient Sanskrit texts.

In fact, we can grasp essential differences between secular and devotional approaches by comparing their metaphysical stances, and also their epistemologies. By this I mean the views of both groups on the kinds of things, beings, or objects that exist; and how, or to what extent, we can know those things, beings, objects.

Devotional scholars claim that there are higher beings, realms, and powers in and beyond the universe. We can know these through yoga meditation, devout study, devotion, and other means. In this view, the purpose of our lives is to attain that higher understanding. Texts such as the *Mahā-bhārata* aim to help us do so.

In contrast, secular scholars tend to believe that such higher beings, realms, and powers either don't exist, or if they do, cannot be objectively verified and are thus not relevant to scholarship. One can thus most reliably and appropriately explain the stories and worlds of the *Mahā-bhārata* in terms of the secular sciences.

More specifically, for several centuries, Western scholars and their acolytes in other regions have repeatedly interpreted India and its culture through the West's protean, historically shifting lenses of ontological and epistemic assumptions.

Early generations of Western Indologists often saw Indian culture through the dogmatic lens of Christian colonialism. As colonialism and Christianity fell out of academic favor in the West, materialistic ideologies rose to replace them. Blown by the winds of academic assumption, and fashion, secular scholars tried to force the *Mahā-bhārata* and other Sanskrit works through a host of secular prisms — Marxist, evolutionist, Freudian, historicist, logical positivist,

---

2 *Stanford Encyclopedia of Philosophy, Aristotle and Metaphysics*

3 To give but one example from the *Bhagavad-gītā*: "I am the source of everything. From me, everything emanates." ahaṃ sarvasya prabhavaḥ mattaḥ sarvaṃ pravartate. [*Gītā* 10.8]

structuralist, feminist, post-colonialist, post-modernist, and many others, mixed and matched to produce endless intellectual flavors.

A common theme of these diverse approaches was that Western-trained scholars understood best the sacred traditions and literature of South Asia. Those inside the tradition were academically impaired by their religious beliefs and could not see the forest for the trees. Thus most secular scholars called the *Mahā-bhārata* mythology. The epic called itself history. Most Western approaches assume that the *Mahā-bhārata*'s descriptions of supernatural beings, powers, or places are mythology, and should be explained in terms of secular approaches, such as psychology, sociology, mythology, and anthropology.

In response, devotional scholars insist that despite its problematic text history, the *Mahā-bhārata* provides its own profound epistemic and interpretive lens, especially in its spiritual core, the celebrated *Bhagavad-gītā*.

To be fair, there have always been secular scholars who strive for strict neutrality, and thus assert that academics should not presume to judge the truth value of claims made by other cultures and their literature. One should rather aim for neutral description, as far as that is possible. Some Western scholars went even further, insisting that cultures and traditions are best grasped through the eyes and voices of those who live inside them.

This wide range of views led to the *insider-outsider* debate within the Western academy. Does the insider, the believer or practitioner, best understand a tradition? Or does the academically trained outsider best understand the ultimate truth of works like the *Mahā-bhārata*? That such debates go on within secular scholarship is a credit to its integrity.

Fortunately, there is a growing recognition among both secular, or *outsider*, scholars and devotional, *insider*, scholars that their different perspectives can be complementary and mutually enriching. We must also give credit to neutral scholars who seek to conscientiously track and document the views of both secular and devotional scholars, thus providing valuable information to all concerned.

I have personally learned from all three — secular, devotional, and neutral scholars. All three groups have aided me in my own work on the *Mahā-bhārata*. I am a devotional *insider* who has benefitted greatly from an excellent outsider education. Good scholarship does not pit believers and non-believers against each other in a zero-sum game. Indeed, both secular and devotional scholars have made enormous contributions to our understanding of the *Mahā-bhārata*, in fields such as archeology, linguistics, philology, history, political and social science, literature, philosophy and theology, and religious studies. The gifts of both groups have been legion. And if I succeed in my purpose, readers of many worldviews will enjoy the story I seek to tell in this work.

Indeed, various visions of this epic story existed even in ancient times when the events reputedly took place! We find evidence of this in another sacred ancient history that describes the same period and many of the same events — the highly revered *Bhāgavata-purāṇa*, also known simply as the *Bhāgavatam*, which at times gives a different version of events found also in the *Mahā-bhārata*. I have used the *Bhāgavatam* extensively, along with the *Mahā-bhārata*, in my attempt to understand this history.

The *Bhāgavatam* claims that when Kṛṣṇa appeared long ago as the central character of the *Bhāgavatam* and the *Mahā-bhārata*, different people had different beliefs about his ultimate identity.

For instance, "…sages experienced Kṛṣṇa as absolute spiritual bliss; those devoted to his service saw Kṛṣṇa as the highest deity; those deep in illusion saw him as an ordinary man; and in their youth, those with great piety played with the child Kṛṣṇa."[4]

Similarly, "When Kṛṣṇa entered the wrestling arena with his older brother, the wrestlers saw him as a thunderbolt; men saw him as an excellent man; women saw him as Cupid incarnate; the cowherd men saw him as one of their own; wicked kings saw him as a punisher; his parents saw him as their child; the Bhoja ruler saw him as death; the unwise as a mere ruler; the yogīs as the highest category of truth; the Vṛṣṇi clan as their highest deity."[5]

Thus, the *Bhāgavatam* assures us that even when Kṛṣṇa lived in our world, some people saw him as a unique spiritual being, others as a human being with special abilities. There have always been insider and outsider views of Kṛṣṇa, who appears prominently in the *Mahā-bhārata* and the *Bhāgavatam*.

---

4 itthaṁ satāṁ brahma-sukhānubhūtyā dāsyaṁ gatānāṁ para-daivatena
māyāśritānāṁ nara-dārakeṇa sākaṁ vijahruḥ kṛta-puṇya-puñjāḥ [BP 10.12.11]

5 mallānām aśanir nṛṇāṁ nara-varaḥ strīṇāṁ smaro mūrtimān
gopānāṁ sva-jano 'satāṁ kṣiti-bhujāṁ śāstā sva-pitroḥ śiśuḥ
mṛtyur bhoja-pater virāḍ aviduṣāṁ tattvaṁ paraṁ yogināṁ
vṛṣṇīnāṁ para-devateti vidito raṅgaṁ gataḥ sāgrajaḥ [BP 10.43.17]

We could say that today, in one sense, we are all outsiders to an ancient culture with values and norms quite different from our own. The devoted will reply that beneath the surface of different cultures, there are eternal spiritual truths intrinsic to the soul. So, changing customs are mere external vehicles to express unchanging spiritual truths in different times and places. Seen apart from their spiritual content and purpose, ancient external cultures may well appear to us as strange and nonrational.

I have spoken of secular and devotional scholarship. Most of us are reasonably familiar with the basic assumptions and methodologies of the secular approach, and the inductive analysis it spawns and regulates. Therefore, we will take a closer look at some of the basic assumptions and methodologies of devotional scholarship. I will begin with my simple analogy of the ant and the arm.

Imagine that a harmless ant is crawling on your forearm. In one sense, the ant knows far more than you about your arm's terrain, as it precisely navigates every freckle and hair, every groove and bump. However, the ant has no idea that your arm even is an arm, or that it belongs to a human person, or what a human person is. Similarly, physical science has achieved a wonderfully precise knowledge of reality's physical surface. But it cannot grasp the multi-dimensional reality beyond that surface. Only in higher states of consciousness can we behold the ultimate reality of life and our place in it. Like the ant navigating your arm, empirical investigations are confined to the surface dimension of a multi-dimensional universe.[6]

My late friend, the brilliant scientist Richard Thompson, gave us another analogy to illustrate the same epistemic point. A man heads to an office located at 10 Main Street. Arriving at that address, he enters the building and searches every door, but cannot find the office. He doesn't know that he is on the ground floor of a multi-story building. The office he seeks is indeed at 10 Main Street, but on a higher floor.

Similarly, the *Bhagavad-gītā* teaches that spiritual practice is like a cognitive elevator that lifts us to higher levels of awareness. There we can perceive higher dimensions of reality, not merely its surface.

---

6 The arm-ant analogy occurred to me one day while sitting on a sandy path on a north Florida farm, New Raman Reti, near Gainesville. An ant actually did crawl on my arm, inspiring the analogy!

From the devotional perspective, why does empirical science necessarily bump up against unyielding cognitive barriers? Because the empirical method requires controlled observation and controlled experiment. Thus, by its own rules, the empirical method can only study an object to the degree that a scientist controls access to, or manipulation of, the object under study. This method, logically, cannot study those aspects of our universe that are knowable, but beyond our control. The fundamental error of dogmatic empiricism is to assume, a priori, that we can only know what we can control.[7]

Coming from, and helping to fashion, the ancient culture that developed yoga and deep meditation, the *Mahā-bhārata* claims that we can know a larger and richer reality — not by trying to control it, but by opening our minds and hearts to life's higher dimensions. We thus directly experience a higher nature so beautiful, sublime, and real that to doubt it becomes self-evidentially irrational, indeed absurd. The *Bhāgavatam* famously focuses even more intensely on the methods and results of profound spiritual meditation. For its part, the empirical method has led to amazing discoveries that greatly improve human life when applied wisely. This method also provides us the sheer intellectual satisfaction of unraveling the fantastic engineering of our world, from the micro to the cosmic.

However, great discoveries, whether physical or metaphysical, often bestow power, power tends to bring pride, and pride can make one foolish. This is true whether the deluded party is a scientist or a priest. Thus, we should try to approach this great epic with an open mind.

The *Mahā-bhārata* has held South Asia spellbound for thousands of years. Thus, we would do well to approach the epic with an open mind. In doing so, we might assume that the epic is a single, ancient text, available to us today. However, that is not exactly the case.

Therefore, we will now consider textual problems that complicate our attempt to understand the *Mahā-bhārata*. Naturally, secular and devotional scholars have different ways of approaching and resolving these problems.

---

7 The empiricist equation, knowable = controllable, entails circular reasoning and self-contradiction, and so is not a logically valid equation. This was one fatal flaw of logical empiricism, also known as logical positivism. Most academic philosophers therefore abandoned it many decades ago.

Within the *Mahā-bhārata* itself, we find a clear recognition of the difficulty of transmitting a teaching over an extended time period. Importantly, this admission occurs in the sacred core of the epic, the *Bhagavad-gītā*. In the fourth chapter, Kṛṣṇa tells Arjuna, "I taught this unperishing Yoga [spiritual science] to Vivasvān, who told it to [his son] Manu. Manu spoke it to [his son] Ikṣvāku. Royal-sages thus learned it as received in [disciplic] succession. After great time in this world, [the spiritual teaching] was lost. Today, I speak to you this same ancient Yoga, this most confidential understanding, for you are My devotee and friend."[8]

Kṛṣṇa affirms that a teaching may be lost or damaged over time. One may recover the original knowledge by hearing from a person who knows it. This principle itself is quite simple and common in our lives. The method, however, takes on greater weight and complexity when the subject matter is the ultimate truth of the universe.

Implicit in Kṛṣṇa's words is the notion that there is an eternal truth that appears and disappears in time, much like the sun that rises and sets to our vision, but always exists.

We may assume here that Kṛṣṇa is not promising to his listener Arjuna that he will restore to his student a precise literal text, in the way that a modern textual scholar would try to reconstruct a lost text. Rather, Kṛṣṇa is eternally cognizant of eternal truth, and he will now teach what he has always known.

Despite the strong spiritual deductive method, so distinct from modern scholarship, we do find here a clear, ancient awareness that teachings can be corrupted or lost over time. For now, it is this that interests us.

Echoing and expanding Kṛṣṇa's statement in the *Bhagavad-gītā*, the celebrated devotional scholar Madhvācārya (1238–1317) saw pervasive text corruptions in the *Mahā-bhārata*, long before Western scholars studied it. In his book, *Mahā-bhārata-tātparya-nirṇaya* (*Ascertaining the Meaning of Mahā-bhārata*), he wrote, "In some parts [of the work], they [scribes or reciters] add texts; in some parts, they even remove texts; in some parts, they carelessly transpose texts; and

---

8 4.1 śrī-bhagavān uvāca
imaṃ vivasvate yogaṃ proktavān aham avyayam
vivasvān manave prāha manur ikṣvākave 'bravīt
4.2 evaṃ paramparā-prāptam imaṃ rājarṣayo viduḥ
sa kāleneha mahatā yogo naṣṭaḥ parantapa
4.3 sa evāyaṃ mayā te 'dya yogaḥ proktaḥ purātanaḥ
bhakto 'si me sakhā ceti rahasyaṃ hy etad uttamam [*Bhagavad-gītā* 4.1-3]

in some parts, they do otherwise. Even texts that are not lost are disordered. [Corruptions occur] throughout." [2.3-4][9]

Modern secular scholars agree that we are dealing with a corrupt text, though they draw very different conclusions from that fact, as I will explain. Before going deeper into that topic, I will outline some likely reasons for the present state of the text.

South Asian tradition gives a very ancient date for the composition of the *Mahā-bhārata* as an unwritten oral tradition. If this is true, for untold centuries, bards and sages transmitted the work orally. It is near impossible to memorize such a huge work. Without a written text, reciters inevitably strayed from the original. Apart from their own human limitations, they often told the stories under heavy political, financial, and sectarian religious pressures. As centuries passed, newer text corruptions built on and overlaid the older ones. Text was inserted. Text was lost. Text was rearranged.

Scholars calculate that roughly 2400 years ago,[10] Sanskrit writing in the Brāhmī script proliferated in India, evolving into the well-known Deva-nāgarī script still used today. As writing became widespread in South Asia, many regional alphabets arose to record various regional languages, and to write classic Sanskrit texts in a regionally legible script. (Even today, most Westerners read Sanskrit verses transliterated into Roman script.) Doubtless, the writing of the *Mahā-bhārata* in many regional scripts dramatically slowed the rate of text corruption, but the damage had been done.

When stories spread orally, and are later written down by diverse people in diverse places, the resultant written texts usually differ significantly. Such was the case with the *Mahā-bhārata*.

---

9 2.3 kvacid granthān prakṣipanti kvacid antaritān api
kuryuḥ kvacic ca vyatyāsaṃ pramādāt kvacid anyathā
2.4 anutsannā api granthā vyākulā iti sarvaśaḥ... [*Mahā-bhārata-tātparya-nirṇaya*]

10 I will not consider here the much older "Indus script", a collection of small seals with raised symbols, produced by the very ancient Indus Valley Civilization, mostly in modern Pakistan and Northwest India. Despite various claims to have deciphered these seals, there is no scholarly consensus supporting any of these claims. We don't really know if the seals depict a language. We have no bilingual inscription to decipher the seals.

In the twentieth century, inspired by successful efforts to discern the original versions of ancient Greco-Roman literature and the *New Testament*, prominent Sanskritists from India, Europe, and America deployed the same scholarly techniques to identify the original text of the *Mahā-bhārata*. Yet here, assiduous scholarly effort fell short.

The Sanskrit Department of Brown University describes this endeavor as follows. "The Critical Edition of...*The Mahābhārata*...[in] 19 vols. (Pune: Bhandarkar Oriental Institute, 1933-1966), [was a] massive editorial project which recorded the readings of hundreds of manuscripts and other forms of testimony from all over the Indian sub-continent and Indonesia. Begun in 1919..., this edition was fundamentally shaped and guided by [Vishnu] Sukthankar, who laid out his editorial map in his brilliant Prolegamena [Introduction] to the first volume of the edition.

"The project was controversial from the beginning: Several scholars have argued that the Mahābhārata textual tradition is too complex, too rooted in living, oral traditions, to be amenable to edition on the basis of principles developed in the more simple literary traditions of Western texts...This [critical edition] is the basis of most contemporary Western scholarship on the Mahābhārata, but at the same time few such scholars, if any, take the critical edition simply at face value."

To better understand what the problems were, let us hear from the critical edition's lead scholar himself, Viṣṇu Sukthankar. All quotes are taken from his renowned Prolegamena, the copious Introduction to this multi-volume work.

After years of prodigious scholarship, Sukthankar threw up his hands, declaring that academic research could not retrieve the epic's original text. "To prevent misconception in the mind of the casual reader, it is best to state at first what the constituted text is *not*. [I am] firmly convinced that the text presented in this edition is *not* anything like the autograph copy of the work of its mythical author, Maharṣi Vyāsa. It is *not*, in any sense, a reconstruction of the *Ur* [original]-*Mahābhārata*..., that ideal but *impossible* desideratum...It is but a modest attempt to present *a version of the epic as old as the extant material will allow us to reach* with some semblance of confidence." [Prolegamena ciii] Similarly, "It is useless to think of reconstructing a...text in a *literally original shape*,...Our objective can only be to reconstruct the oldest form of the text which it is possible to reach on the basis of the manuscript material available." [Prolegamena vxxxvi]

Sukthankar even seems to imply that there never was an original text! He urges upon his readers, "…this essential fact in Mahābhārata textual criticism, that the *Mahābhārata* is not and *never was* a fixed rigid text, but is fluctuating epic tradition…" [Prolegamena cii]

Ultimately, Sukthankar tried to see the sunny side of the failure to find an original text within a sea of *spurious additions*. "When I say that the Mahābhārata manuscripts contain quantities of spurious additions, I intend no disparagement or condemnation of the text or of the manuscripts. The process [of text corruption] is normal, inevitable, and in a wider sense *wholly right* [my emphasis]. *If* the epic is to continue to be a vital force in the life of any progressive people, *it must be a slow-changing book*! Thus, a progressive people need a progressively evolving book." [Prolegamena ci]

Van Buitenen, the first scholar to attempt, and partially complete, a translation of the *Mahā-bhārata*'s critical edition, made a similar point. "Unlike the Vedas, which have to be preserved letter-perfect, the epic was a popular work whose reciters would inevitably conform to changes in language and style."[20] Buitenen (1973) pp. xxiv–xxv

Devotional scholars like Madhvācārya acknowledged the *spurious* additions in the text seven centuries before modern scholars did so. If anything, Madhvācārya is more severe in his assessment of the text. But he and other devotional scholars insist that there is indeed an original story, and that story is ultimately history, events that really took place long, long ago on this planet.

As we saw, the ancient *Bhagavad-gītā* speaks openly of problems in text transmission. The *Bhagavad-gītā* is part of the *Mahā-bhārata*. Thus, the epic itself warns that teachings tend to be adulterated over time. Further, neither Kṛṣṇa nor Madhvācarya opposes the speaking of an ancient teaching in contemporary language. Both do precisely that. But the essential message and story must be preserved. That is what did not happen in the case of the *Mahā-bhārata*.

Sukthankar saw positive elements in the text's "evolution" over time. Additions, changes, and removals of text merely contemporized a literary centerpiece of South Asian civilization.

In contrast, Madhvācārya only sees the loss and corruption of an invaluable, original, sacred history. This is not valuable, adaptive evolution in action, as Sukthankar suggests, but rather a tragic loss. In that, Madhvācārya echoes

Kṛṣṇa's claim in the *Bhagavad-gītā* that his original pure spiritual teaching perished over great time, implying that this fact is related to the loss of virtue and justice in the world.[11]

Kṛṣna, in the *Gītā*, is restoring his original message by teaching it to Arjuna. Madhvācārya similarly claims that *by divine mercy*, he will restore the original meaning of the *Mahā-bhārata*.[12] Thus he wrote, "Although the text is thus disordered, and its meaning is hard for even gods to approach, when things are thus confused in the [fallen] Kali age, inspired by Lord Hari to [discern] the [real] conclusions, I shall speak the conclusions, understanding them by His mercy, and knowing also other *śāstras* [scriptures] and the *Vedas* by His mercy."[13]

Madhvācārya claims to restore the original meaning not by text-critical scholarship, but rather by divine revelation. Still, despite these stark differences in restorative methodologies, secular and devotional scholars do agree on the present state of the text.

But how old is the *Mahā-bhārata*? Even if we cannot recover an original text, can we say when that text might have been composed? How should we interpret Sukthankar's claim of an "...essential fact in *Mahābhārata* textual criticism, that the *Mahābhārata* is not and *never was* a fixed rigid text, but is fluctuating epic tradition..." [Prolegamena cii]

Do we have clear evidence to support Sukthankar's rather radical claim? I don't think we do. Here are some related reasons why.

1. We cannot rationally *assume* that the *Mahā-bhārata* is not based on historical events, however imperfectly the surviving text tradition preserved those events. Thus, if a divine Avatāra, Vyāsa, descended to this world and described those real historical events, then the text had a definite beginning as *itihāsa*, history.

2. If all that is true, then eyewitnesses to the history, or those alive at the time who heard from witnesses, passed on what they knew to the next generations. Thus, if the *Mahā-bhārata* was born of history, and preserved by an Avatāra, then

11 *Bhagavad-gītā* 4.7-8

12 Kṛṣṇa's *Bhagavad-gītā* is far more widely accepted than Madhvācārya's treatise on the *Mahā-bhārata*. Within the devotional community, not all restorations of sacred text are seen as equal.

13 2.5 grantho 'py evaṃ vilulitaḥ kim nv artho deva-durgamaḥ
kalāv evaṃ vyākulite nirṇayāya pracoditaḥ
2.6 hariṇā nirṇayān vacmi vijānaṃs tat-prasādataḥ
śāstrāntarāṇi sañjānan vedāṃś cāsya prasādataḥ [*Mahā-bhārata-tātparya-nirṇaya*]

for at least a limited time, the text would probably not expand wildly beyond its original boundaries.

3. Later generations, far more distant from the original events, might be more inclined to embellish, add, subtract, or mythologize. Mythologization might have occurred early on, but the pace could well have accelerated as the original events faded into a remote, legendary past.

4. The fact that the many varying recensions are still today easily recognizable as the same book indicates that corrupting tendencies were moderated by the deep veneration in which most people held the story and its putative author.

If devotional scholars cannot *prove* the historical thesis with all the tools and methods of modern scholarship, neither can secular scholars disprove it. Thus the opposing views do not indicate an opposition of scholarship versus faith, or reason versus unreason, but rather two equally rigorous and internally coherent worldviews built on opposing epistemic and ontological foundations. These in turn depend upon the self-evidential life experiences of each group. By this I mean that one's personal experience of the world influences, and at times even determines, one's choice of methodology. We tend to choose those methodologies that have yielded for us convincing experiences.

Many people, perhaps hundreds of millions in India alone, remain committed to the *Mahā-bhārata* as a source, however problematic, of sacred history. Despite all the epic's textual issues, these many people remain convinced that the great epic still retains a significant amount of historical and spiritual truth. Fortunately for the devoted, they have another, textually more reliable source of sacred history that confirms many, though not all, of the main events recounted in the epic. This source is the legendary *Bhāgavata-purāṇa*, also known simply as the *Bhāgavatam*.

Compared to the *Mahā-bhārata*, the *Bhāgavatam*'s ancient text is relatively uncorrupted and intact. Indeed the text variants listed in the *Bhāgavatam's* critical text are few and inconsequential in comparison to those of the *Mahā-bhārata*. The *Bhāgavatam* contains far more advanced theology and explicitly claims to correct what it considers to be theological and narrative misconceptions in the *Mahā-bhārata*.

I have personally translated and published, with commentaries, 119 chapters of the *Bhāgavatam*. I have regularly consulted and profited from its Sanskrit text in the writing of this book. I have also studied the versions of major events as they are depicted in the other major Purāṇas, many of whose textual integrity does not match that of the *Bhāgavatam*.

Secular scholars will point out that the *Bhāgavatam* appeared on the scene various centuries later than the *Mahā-bhārata*, and thus cannot claim to provide eyewitness accounts, nor testimonies from those somehow related to the epic events.

The *Bhāgavatam* itself replies to these critiques, stating that the Lord personally inspired, and manifests within, the *Bhāgavatam*. Devoted readers experience this fact so powerfully that it becomes for them a *properly basic* epistemic foundation, i.e., a self-evident fact upon which one builds and bases a secure knowledge system.

Here too, we confront two different ways of knowing — secular and devotional. To call the secular way objective, and the devotional way subjective, would betray a serious degree of philosophical naiveté. But let us return to the *Mahā-bhārata*.

DATING THE TEXT

Despite Sukthankar's claim "that the *Mahābhārata* is not and *never* was a fixed rigid text, but is fluctuating epic tradition…", many scholars, secular and devotional, attempt to date the text. I will briefly review a few of those attempts.

I will begin again with Sukthankar, who issues a dating caveat to his critical edition. "The constituted text *cannot be accurately dated*, nor labelled as pertaining to any particular place or personality…It goes without saying that [like every other edition] it is *a mosaic of old and new matter.*"[14] [Prolegamena ciii]

Thus, to date the text, scholars look for *external references*, i.e., datable texts, inscriptions etc. that mention the *Mahā-bhārata*. As respected *Mahā-bhārata* scholar John Brockington states "…the earliest 'surviving' components of this dynamic text are believed to be no older than the earliest 'external' references we have to the epic, which may include an allusion in Pāṇini's 4th century BCE grammar Aṣṭādhyāyī 4:2:56."[15]

---

14 This mixing of text from different historical periods is also found in a similar genre of old Sanskrit literature called Purāṇas, *Ancient History*, dealing with cosmogony, cosmology, royal lines, heroic and didactic histories, and other topics.

15 Brockington, 1998, 26.

Tying the epic's date to *external references* is understandable, but not always reliable. The dates of *external references* are themselves often uncertain. Further, if so much of a culturally central work like the *Mahā-bhārata* was lost, it is far more likely that far less important works *that referred* to the *Mahā-bhārata* also perished. Perhaps most importantly, the problem of dating a text *whose oldest version cannot be found and is probably lost* is obvious.

The conclusion would seem to be that simply by examining and comparing texts, we do not know with certainty how old the *Mahā-bhārata* is. This makes it difficult to glean from the surviving text a precise date for the events described therein, if we suspect them to be roughly historical, and not mere myth. We do have evidence that points to a date of extreme antiquity for the epic. We will consider that now.

The *Aihole inscription*, found in an old Jain temple in Aihole, Karnataka, is dated to 634 CE, during the reign of Pulakeśin II. This inscription states that 3,735 years have passed from the time of the great Kuru-kṣetra war, the climax of the *Mahā-bhārata*, till the time of the inscription, composed by the poet Ravi-kīrti.

I am writing these words in 2022 CE. Therefore, since the time of the Aihole inscription, 1,388 years have passed. Thus the inscription claims that a central event of the *Mahā-bhārata* took place 5,123 years ago, in the year 3101 BCE. We might not pay great attention to this ancient inscription if it did not precisely confirm a date for the *Mahā-bhārata* coming from another, unusually credible source.

The *Mahā-bhārata*, the *Bhāgavatam*, and other ancient Sanskrit literatures often give the positions of stars and planets at the time of important events. The great Indian mathematician and astronomer Arya-bhata (476 - 550 CE), a co-founder of trigonometry, among his many celebrated achievements, studied the epic's descriptions of the positions of planets and stars at the time of major *Mahā-bhārata* events, such as the Kuru-kṣetra War. As one of history's great mathematicians, and a learned astronomer, he then calculated when in the past the night sky would have shown to a human observer the specific celestial configurations described in the epic.

This dating method is sometimes called archaeo-astronomy, or historical astronomy. Arya-bhata concluded from astronomical descriptions in the *Mahā-bhārata* that the Kuru-kṣetra War took place roughly 5,100 years ago. Many Indian and some Western scholars, in various disciplines, support this date and present additional arguments to bolster it. Other Western Indologists argue for a later date.

Arya-bhata concluded that the Kuru-kṣetra War took place in 3102 BCE, or 5,124 years ago, a date nearly identical to that of the Aihole inscription. One may argue that Ravi-kīrti, the author of the Aihole inscription, simply borrowed Arya-bhata's date. However Arya-bhata lived far away from Aihole, in the area of modern Patna, and neither Ravi-kīrti, nor his king, nor anyone else associated with the inscription, mentions Arya-bhata, who died eighty-four years before its creation. In any case, over the centuries, Hindus have widely accepted Arya-bhata's date for the Kuru-kṣetra War, and more generally for the period in which Kṛṣṇa appeared in this world, as described in the *Mahā-bhārata*.

One might think that the ancient culture described in *Mahā-bhārata*, if it truly existed, must have left archeological remains throughout Northern India. But here too, as in critical text studies, secular scholarship cannot definitively adjudicate the historicity of the *Mahā-bhārata*. I will explain why.

We begin with a simple but huge problem plaguing South Asian archeology: very little of South Asia has been seriously excavated. American archaeologist Sarah Parcak of the University of Alabama stated, "I…feel confident saying more than 90% of…[South Asian] archaeological sites have not been excavated…India has such an extraordinary and rich heritage, with many thousands of years of occupation…Thus, I would estimate that more than 90% of India's heritage is [still] buried…"[16]

This problem will not be soon remedied. "Smriti Haricharan [of the] National Institute of Advanced Studies, says archeology remains underfunded [in India] and departments of archaeology are few in number, and understaffed."[17]

The Archeological Survey of India, founded by the British in 1861, is India's central government agency responsible for archeology and the preservation of historical monuments. Beyond its own problems of underfunding and understaffing, difficulties beyond this agency's power make it difficult for archeology to give a definitive picture of India's ancient past. Here are some of the problems.

1. India has suffered brutal invasions that destroyed many ancient and monumental structures

---

16 *Times of India* 28.12.21

17 *Deccan Herald* 12.22.21

2. The population density of India is about four times that of other ancient civilizations such as Mesopotamia and Egypt. Thus far more potential sites have been continually inhabited to this day. So, access is severely limited. Ancient artifacts and structures that do emerge are often repurposed, sold, thrown away, or destroyed.

3. Rapid urbanization in modern India makes a vast and growing number of sites unavailable for excavation.

I repeat Parcak's conclusion. "...I would estimate that more than 90% of India's heritage is buried..."

To vividly grasp the heavy challenges facing Indian archeology, let us consider the case of Rakhigarhi, a village about 85 miles northwest of Delhi, and close to the geographic center of *Mahā-bhārata* events. Rakhigarhi is a high-value archeological site for several reasons. It yielded rare DNA, about 4,500 years old. "It took a massive, time-consuming effort to produce the genome from remains found in the cemetery at Rakhigarhi."[18] Further, Rakhigarhi was a major city of the ancient Indus Valley Civilization, and it lies but 150 kilometers from ancient Indra-prastha, one of the most important cities in the *Mahā-bhārata*.

The Archeological Survey of India began excavating this site in 1963, though little was published. Yet by 2020, almost sixty years later, the ASI and Deccan College had excavated only 5% of the site, according to the daily newspaper *The Hindu*.[19]

In an article dated April 16, 2015, *The Tribune* of India declared, "Lack of official protection and plunder of treasure troves, hidden underneath, by unscrupulous elements are *playing havoc with the 5,000-year-old ancient archaeological site* belonging to the Indus Valley civilization in the village [of Rakhigarhi].

"While a good part of the site had been *destroyed* by soil erosion, encroachments and illegal sand lifting by the farmers is damaging the rest.

"Some villagers told [us] that the antiquities being recovered from the site had been sold for the past many years. There are many people in nearby villages who own antiquities, including domestic terracotta items, copper objects, precious stones, beads, shells etc.

---

18 *Rare Ancient DNA Provides Window Into a 5,000-Year-Old South Asian Civilization*, Brian Handwerk, *Smithsonian Magazine*, September 5, 2019.

19 *The Hindu*, Feb 27, 2020

"Global Heritage Fund (GHF), an international organisation working for protection of endangered sites in the developing world, ...included Rakhigarhi as [one of] Asia's 10 most significant archaeological sites facing *irreparable loss and destruction.*

"'It is one of the largest and oldest Indus sites in the world which is facing threat due to development pressures, insufficient management and looting', the GHF report mentions."[20]

With all these problems, what archeological information do we actually have about India in the approximate time and locations of the *Mahā-bhārata*? From 1950 to 1952, B.B. Lal, who later served as Archeological Survey of India director, focused on archeological sites related to events in the *Mahā-bhārata*, such as Hastinapur, the great royal capital of the Kurus. Lal was inclined to see the stories of the *Mahā-bhārata*, and its sister epic, the *Rāmāyaṇa*, as based on historical events.

In 1952, Lal began excavations at Hastinapur. He found some ancient remains, such as elegant grey pottery painted with black geometric patterns, dated to as early as 1300 BCE. This pottery has been found in over 1,100 sites extending over a wide area, and is linked to village and town sites, domesticated horses, ivory-working, and the advent of iron metallurgy.

Later, somewhat older black and red ware pottery was found. Clearly, we can draw no detailed conclusions from this, since we do not have evidence as to exactly who made this pottery, and what their possible relation was to the *Mahā-bhārata* culture. As I often heard Dr. Witzel say in classes at Harvard, "Pots don't speak."

After a hiatus of nearly 70 years, the ASI is again planning to do serious excavations at Hastinapur. "The plan is to look for new evidence to ground the 'Mahabharata' in history and preserve earlier finds."[21]

Other recent archeological efforts also seek to correlate findings with the *Mahā-bhārata*, such as the excavations at Lakshagriha.[22] To be precise, we do not definitely know that the current Indian town of Hastinapur , the focal point of archeological efforts, is in fact the ancient Kuru capital of Hastinā-pura. The *Mahā-bhārata* itself states that the Ganges River rose and swept away the ancient city.

---

20 *The Tribune India*, Apr 16, 2015

21 *The Times of India*, Jul 20, 2021

22 "The Lakshagriha Excavation Project," *Hindustan Times*, April 8, 2018

Nor do we know with certainty that other sites of similar interest precisely correspond to places mentioned in the epic.

Another *Mahā-bhārata* site which has raised keen interest is the area around the modern city of Dwarka on the west coast of Gujarat, believed to be the site of Kṛṣṇa's fabled island city of Dvārakā.

From 1983 to 1990, the Marine Archaeology Unit of India's National Institute of Oceanography (NIO) carried out underwater excavations at Dwarka and Bet Dwarka, in search of Kṛṣṇa's city. The *Mahā-bhārata* and other sacred texts claim that when Kṛṣṇa and his associates left this world, the sea level rose, submerging the city in the Arabian Sea.

According to a UNESCO report, "Between 1983 and 1990 the archaeologists discovered a fortified foundation on which the ancient city walls must have been built along the river banks. Stone blocks used for the construction, pillars and irrigation systems were found but a debate is still ongoing regarding the dating of the vestiges, either from 3,000 to 1,500 years BC or from the Middle Ages."[23]

Though fascinating and suggestive, these studies do not prove beyond doubt, and certainly do not disprove, that we have recovered material evidence of the culture and events described in the *Mahā-bhārata*. Just as "pots don't speak," sadly, neither do submerged stone blocks and pillars. As at Hastinā-pura, no one has recovered at these sites clear, ancient textual proof to identify them. Again, by the strict standards of secular scholarship, we simply do not know who carved the blocks and placed the pillars at Dwarka.

DNA AND AGRICULTURE

I will end my brief survey of South Asian archeology with a word on ancient agriculture, a probable indicator of a developed culture. At issue here is whether ancient South Asian agriculture, and the culture it sustained, were indigenous to South Asia. Or did they come from outside, from ancient Mesopotamia, or from Indo-European peoples that conquered, migrated to, or civilized the indigenous people of South Asia?

Although scholars previously believed "that agriculture arrived in the Indo-Pakistani region via migration from the Fertile Crescent of the Middle East,

---

23 https://en.unesco.org/silkroad/silk-road-themes/underwater-heritage/dwarka

the ancient Harappan genes show little contribution from that lineage, suggesting that farming spread through an exchange of ideas rather than a mass migration, or perhaps even arose independently in South Asia. ... [T]he first farmers of the Fertile Crescent appear to have contributed little, genetically, to South Asian populations. '...similar practices of farming are present in South Asia by about 8,000 B.C. or so,' says Priya Moorjani, a population geneticist at UC Berkeley."[24]

How is all this relevant to our discussion of the *Mahā-bhārata*? It seems that North and Northwest India, key regions in the epic, did not import from the Middle East culture that is crucial to *Mahā-bhārata* events. Rather, the area associated with the epic developed its own advanced culture. This agrees with the self-understanding of the *Mahā-bhārata*.

GRAVE SITES

Archeology often depends on the excavation of grave sites to learn of ancient cultures. In that sense too, South Asian archeology could well be hampered. For comparison, Egyptian rulers constructed monumental funerary pyramids, replete with ancient cultural items and text engravings. These items have played an essential role in our broad understanding of ancient Egypt.

In stark contrast, the *Mahā-bhārata* everywhere describes a culture of cremation. No text, no funerary items, and thus little understanding of the ancient culture.

ANCIENT TEXTS

As described earlier, the *Mahā-bhārata* depicts an oral society. If, even hypothetically, we use the dates given by Aryabhata and the Aihole inscription, then the events so vividly described in the epic took place thousands of years before translatable writing appeared in South Asia. Thus archeologists will likely look in vain for ancient inscriptions, texts, or epigraphs that explain archeological findings.

Conclusion: the material conditions in India severely limit the power of archeology and related disciplines to reveal with certainty the historicity of

24 *Rare Ancient DNA Provides Window Into a 5,000-Year-Old South Asian Civilization*, Brian Handwerk, *Smithsonian Magazine*, September 5, 2019.

people, events, and conditions depicted in ancient Sanskrit literature such as the *Mahā-bhārata* and the *Bhāgavatam*.

MY APPROACH

As my main sources, I have relied on the critical Sanskrit text of the *Mahā-bhārata*, which provides the most complete record possible of known text variants. I have also regularly consulted Vettam Mani's well-known *Purāṇic Encyclopedia*, which explains how important characters in the epic were depicted in the eighteen major Purāṇas and other ancient Sanskrit texts. I paid special attention to the famous *Bhāgavatam*, which I have already described, and which occupies a unique position in the tradition, both in spiritual and literary terms.

My presentation of this ancient story does not require the reader to hold a particular worldview. I hope that all kinds of readers will keep an open mind and enjoy the story.

My approach to the text is both critical and devotional. I agree with devotional scholars such as the 13th-century Madhvācārya, and with most modern scholars, that the Sanskrit texts of the *Mahā-bhārata* available to us today are seriously corrupted versions of the original. So, a literal translation of the surviving texts, or a summary of them, would not fulfill my dream of reconstructing, or one might even say reimagining, as far as possible, the original story.

I am keenly aware of how pretentious or impractical my dream will appear to some, both on cross-cultural and spiritual grounds. Some will reject my ability, or any contemporary person's ability, to deeply understand an ancient culture so far removed from us by time and custom. However, in my view, we must not be confused by major differences in the surface culture of their world and ours. Beneath that surface we discover not only a universal humanity, but explicitly a story of souls, a story that all souls in all times can understand if they will open their hearts and minds to it. Kṛṣṇa himself teaches that clear knowledge sees unity in diversity, the universal within the particular.[25]

---

25 sarva-bhūteṣu yenaikaṃ bhāvam avyayam īkṣate
avibhaktaṃ vibhakteṣu taj jñānaṃ viddhi sāttvikam Bg 18.20

I confess that fifty-three years of disciplined practice within the primary spiritual tradition of the *Bhagavad-gītā* have convinced me that serious attention to the geopolitical and human reality of the epic, as well as to its clear, overarching spiritual narrative, can indeed enable us to excavate in its broad outline something like the original story. Rather than argue for my understanding, I will leave it to each reader to consult their own mind and heart about the plausibility of the story you are about to read.

Apart from that claim, which I know will leave some incredulous, what is special or unique about this version of an endlessly told tale? Here are a few ways in which this version may be somewhat unique.

1. The many translations and adaptations of the epic, in whole or in parts, seem to adopt one of two approaches. The *outsider*, such as the skeptical, secular scholar, sees mainly myth and fable. The faithful *insider* sees and presents the epic story chiefly as history, even when such authors change or reimagine some details of character and plot.

I am an *insider* who accepts unbiased evidence from both secular and devotional scholars. I seek to excavate an original history by examining all important events through the philosophical lens of the *Bhagavad-gītā*, and the corrective narrative lens of the *Bhāgavatam*. Within this framework, I seek to apply rigorous historical analysis. The specific method and the result are somewhat unique.

2. Previous translations, summaries, and reimaginings of the *Mahā-bhārata* tend to focus on the fifth generation of the central narrative, the generation in which Kṛṣṇa, the five Pāṇḍava brothers, Duryodhana, Karṇa, etc., all appear. However, following an ancient option mentioned in the epic itself,[26] I begin with the reign of King Vasu of Cedi, four generations before those central characters. I find this essential to fully grasp the historical context in which the most famous events unfold.

3. I follow another ancient option by omitting the epic's secondary stories (*upākhyāna*-s) which do not directly bear on the main story, yet strikingly make up around 80% of the unabridged text![27] I believe that for my purpose, this superfluity of marginal material disrupts the flow and momentum of the central

---

26 Verse 1.1.50 of the criticial edition: "some sages begin their careful study of the text with the story of King Uparicara Vasu." *tathoparicarādy anye viprāḥ samyag adhīyate*

27 *The Britannica*, in its article on the epic, remarks that "The central plot constitutes little more than one fifth of the total work. The remainder...addresses a wide range of myths and legends."

narrative. Some ancient reciters and audiences also felt this way, for the *Mahā-bhārata* itself refers to a shorter, abridged version with four times fewer verses, and without the secondary stories.[28]

4. I also seek to address in my work a rather curious phenomenon—modern attempts to "correct" the text that in my view actually take us farther away from the text's original meaning. These distortions of the main story and characters arise both in the devotional community and among secular scholars. I will give but one example of distortion, among many, within both Hindu and secular communities. I begin in the Hindu realm.

The central character in my first volume is the brilliant young lady Satya-vatī (pronounced Satya-vatee), whom I greatly admire. Contrary to what we find in the critical Sanskrit text, many Hindus have come to see Satya-vatī as a lady of rather terrible character.

We find one of many examples of this in an uncontested Wikipedia article on Satya-vatī [spelled there Satyavati]. "While Satyavati's...mastery of realpolitik is praised, her *unscrupulous* means of achieving her goals and her *blind ambition* are criticized [by many Hindus].

"Dhanalakshmi Ayyer, author of *Satyavati: Blind Ambition*, claims that Satyavati's '...motherly ambition [blinds] her vision at every turn.'

"For Satyavati the end matters, not the means...Her actions (and decisions) create a generation encompassed by a greed..."

What is perhaps most interesting about these unchallenged public insults to Satya-vatī is that none of them, not one, finds a source or basis in the critical text of the *Mahā-bhārata* itself. Confident Hindu critics, of which there are many, forget that Satya-vatī, far from being a selfish, scheming materialistic woman, is the mother of a major Avatāra. She was chosen to play a leading role in rescuing our planet because of her divine qualities. We observe here how those within a sacred tradition can drift from their sacred texts and slander their own great matriarchs.

But the privilege of gratuitous criticism extends equally to those outside the faith tradition. I cite here one example from an esteemed scholar who often contributed valuable insights. The late J.A.B. van Buitenen of the University of

---

28 1.1.61 catur-viṃśati-sāhasrīṃ cakre bhārata-saṃhitām
upākhyānair vinā tāvad bhārataṃ procyate budhaiḥ

Chicago, was the first scholar to begin a translation of the *Mahā-bhārata*'s critical text, completing three volumes before his unfortunate demise.

In the Introduction to his first volume, the *Ādi-parva*, or *first book*, van Buitenen made a scathing criticism of a key theme of the sacred narration — the descent of Avatāras, superhuman entities, both good and evil, who appeared on Earth as apparent human beings, using our planet as a type of cosmic battleground. A long list of these descents, in the epic's first book, Chapter 61, garnered van Buitenen's special disdain.

He declared this central *Mahā-bhārata* theme to be "...*decadent* sanctification by mythology." Moreover, it is "*inept* mythification...decaying mythology,... needlessly presented...and best ignored." It is "inane," which in my dictionary means *silly and stupid*. [JAB xx-xxi]

Yet much of what this scholar saw as *decadent, needless, inane, inept,* and *best ignored* has struck countless devoted listeners and readers, for dozens of centuries, as thrilling and deeply meaningful. Indeed the descent of Kṛṣṇa to this world, his fight for justice against superhuman foes, and his speaking of *Bhagavad-gītā* on a climactic battlefield, stand at the center of Indian self-understanding.

Even if, for whatever reason, one rejects the spiritual claims of the epic, the general theme of interplanetary battles between earthlings and aliens disguised as earthlings constitutes one of Hollywood's most popular genres. Clearly, the human mind is deeply, perhaps intuitively, receptive to, and fascinated by, this idea. Thus, whether one takes this *Mahā-bhārata* theme as real history, or as mere epic storytelling, it has powerfully connected with deep human intuition and dramatic taste. It does not deserve all the scorn heaped upon it by numerous scholars. And of course a secular scholar ultimately can have no idea, *in his or her role as a secular scholar*, whether such extraterrestrial battles actually took place or not. I have utilized what I consider to be good scholarship, whatever its source, and passed on mere skepticism posing as neutral scholarship.

5. Sadly, I must agree with both devotional and secular scholars that the surviving recensions of the *Mahā-bhārata* display clear and numerous text corruptions. Thus, even for the faithful, the surviving text itself impedes our understanding of an original sacred history.

Among various discernible categories of text corruption, I will here focus on only one, since it specifically weakens the epic's ability to attract modern readers. I define this problem as *narrative amnesia*. The mere 20% of the text that tells the main story more often than not forgets the overarching theme powerfully presented at the beginning — the invasion of Earth and the battle to save it.

Kṛṣṇa emphasizes this central theme in two of the *Bhagavad-gītā*'s most famous verses, wherein he explains exactly why he came to this world in the first place.

"Whenever justice fails and injustice prevails, I myself appear. [4.7] To deliver the righteous and vanquish the wicked, and to restore justice, I appear in every age." [4.8][29]

The *Bhāgavatam* itself strongly criticizes the *Mahā-bhārata* for neglecting this central theme.[30] The problem, from this perspective, is not as van Buitenen claims, that a human story was polluted with *inane* and *inept* mythic overlays of Avatāras descending to Earth. The problem is exactly the opposite, as the *Bhāgavatam* points out— an amazing spiritual and cosmic story was shrunk into mundane human proportions.

As I worked on this book, I happily discovered that the central theme, if kept central, sheds dazzling light on many parts of the story that have long confused readers. So, as presumptuous and improbable as it may sound to some, this book is an earnest, painstaking attempt to correct centuries of textual and extra-textual corruption, the latter coming from both inside and outside the sacred tradition.

6. My rendition of this ancient story assumes that it is possible to connect with, and deeply grasp, people and events that took place long ago in a faraway land. Naturally some will deny the possibility of anyone today fully or deeply understanding an ancient culture so different from our own.

To justify my attempt, at least theoretically, I appeal again to Kṛṣṇa in the *Bhagavad-gītā*. Kṛṣṇa explicitly addresses the issue of whether one can legitimately perceive universal principles behind a variegated surface. In fact, one can. Here is Kṛṣṇa's statement.

---

29 4.7 yadā yadā hi dharmasya glānir bhavati bhārata
abhyutthānam adharmasya tadātmānaṃ sṛjāmy aham
4.8 paritrāṇāya sādhūnāṃ vināśāya ca duṣkṛtām
dharma-saṃsthāpanārthāya sambhavāmi yuge yuge

30 *Bhāgavata-pūrāṇa* 1.5.8-9,15

"True, essential knowledge perceives a single unperishing reality in all beings, undivided within the divided. [Bg 18.20] Know that it is hazy knowledge that perceives various beings of different types as fundamentally different." [Bg 18.21][31]

With the term *hazy knowledge* (rājasaṃ jñānam), Kṛṣṇa describes a state in which our clear consciousness is covered or obscured. Eight times in the *Bhagavad-gītā*, Kṛṣṇa uses various forms of the verb *āvṛ*, *to cover*, *hide*, *conceal*, to explain how material illusion *covers* our pure consciousness. For example, in verses 3.38-40, Kṛṣṇa states, "As smoke *covers* fire, as dust *covers* a mirror, and the womb *covers* the embryo, so is this world covered. The knowledge of the knower is *covered* by his or her eternal enemy in the form of material desire, which, like fire, cannot be quenched. The senses, mind, and reason are its abode. By *covering* spiritual knowledge, this [material desire] bewilders the embodied soul."[32]

The *Bhagavad-gītā* uses the same verb, *āvṛ*, in five other verses to explain the same point — material desires cover our pure awareness.[33] Consider the simple analogy of a traffic light which alternately shows red, yellow, and green light. In fact, behind the red, yellow, and green *coverings* is the same white or pure light. Similarly, within the soul is pure consciousness. When that pure consciousness passes through a body, the consciousness takes on the body's qualities in terms of race, gender, age, ethnicity, species, inclination, etc. To understand spiritual

---

31 sarva-bhūteṣu yenaikaṃ bhāvam avyayam īkṣate
avibhaktaṃ vibhakteṣu taj jñānaṃ viddhi sāttvikam 18.20
pṛthaktvena tu taj jñānaṃ nānā-bhāvān pṛthag-vidhān
vetti sarveṣu bhūteṣu taj jñānaṃ viddhi rājasam 18.21

32 dhūmenāvriyate vahnir yathādarśo malena ca
yatholbenāvṛto garbhas tathā tenedam āvṛtam 3.38
āvṛtaṃ jñānam etena jñānino nitya-vairiṇā
kāma-rūpeṇa kaunteya duṣpūreṇānalena ca 3.39
indriyāṇi mano buddhir asyādhiṣṭhānam ucyate
etair vimohayaty eṣa jñānam āvṛtya dehinam 3.40

33 nādatte kasyacit pāpaṃ na caiva sukṛtaṃ vibhuḥ
ajñānenāvṛtaṃ jñānaṃ tena muhyanti jantavaḥ 5.15
nāhaṃ prakāśaḥ sarvasya yoga-māyā-samāvṛtaḥ
mūḍho 'yaṃ nābhijānāti loko mām ajam avyayam 7.25
sattvaṃ sukhe sañjayati rajaḥ karmaṇi bhārata
jñānam āvṛtya tu tamaḥ pramāde sañjayaty uta 14.9
aneka-citta-vibhrāntā moha-jāla-samāvṛtāḥ
prasaktāḥ kāma-bhogeṣu patanti narake 'sucau 16.16
adharmaṃ dharmam iti yā manyate tamasāvṛtā
sarvārthān viparītāṃś ca buddhiḥ sā pārtha tāmasī 18.32

knowledge, one must find the pure nature and awareness of oneself and others, beyond bodily filters. It is precisely that pure awareness, consciousness, that unites all souls in all times and places.

Interestingly, we find a clear analogy to this form of reasoning in the world of empirical science. Indeed, in trying to deeply understand the characters in the story, I have applied a basic principle of physical science to a metaphysical story, finding that it works equally well in both dimensions. I shall explain.

First developed in geology in the late 18th century, the *doctrine of uniformity* claims that nature's laws, i.e., physical cause and effect, function uniformly throughout space-time. That is, the same physical laws govern all times and places in the physical universe.

The *Bhagavad-gītā* teaches that there are uniform metaphysical laws that govern all times and places of our universe. These laws do not oppose free will, but rather respond rationally and reciprocally to our free choices. Just as our bodies activate and respond to uniform physical laws, so as conscious, metaphysical beings, we activate and respond to metaphysical laws that morally govern the universe.

Souls are not identical in every sense. That would make for a dull universe. Each soul is unique, but all souls are endowed with equal ethical and epistemic *competence*. Thus each soul is responsible for its decisions and choices. The *Bhagavad-gītā* describes this uniform responsibility of souls, and the universe's uniform response to their choices, in a single word — *karma*.

Science cannot *prove* the uniformity of physical laws, certainly not in faraway places and times. But consistent, predictable results are taken to confirm the principle. Metaphysical science, if we use the term, would logically require a different method to confirm results. Nonetheless, both physical and metaphysical science rely on clear confirmation within the consciousness of the observer. Physical science, as stated earlier, requires us to control phenomena, by controlling access to, observation of, and manipulation of physical things. This method, by its own rules, limits the scientist to the study of objects that are in principle inferior to us, in that we can control them.

Metaphysical science seeks to study that which is greater than us. This rules *out* empirical methodologies that require control over the objects to be studied. The *Bhagavad-gītā* presents a metaphysical science that has convinced and enlightened very large numbers of human beings, over very long timespans. Clearly many people do not understand this science, just as most people do not personally understand advanced physical science.

A sustained discussion of this issue awaits a more suitable context. For now, I only mention the fundamental principles that underlie the worldview of the wisest participants in the epic action of the *Mahā-bhārata.* I will now conclude this introduction, lest it grow beyond reasonable proportion.

I have shown that secular scholarship cannot recover an original *Mahā-bhārata*, and even if it could, it does not have the power to discern the ultimate historicity of the text, and much less the truth of its metaphysical claims. What about devotional scholarship?

I have spent fifty-three years immersed in an ancient bhakti-yoga tradition which in its broad outlines is the spiritual center of this epic tale. I have personally translated from the original Sanskrit hundreds of chapters of both the *Mahā-bhārata* and the *Bhāgavatam*, my two principal sources.

I would be disingenuous were I not to disclose my conviction that spiritual communication is possible across time and *cultures*, and that my version of a sacred ancient story has much in its favor. Each reader must judge for themself whether this story rings true for them, and to what extent.

In his Foreword to a *Bhāgavatam* volume that he generously financed, Beatle George Harrison urged Western readers to give this literature and its worldview a chance, concluding that "The proof of the pudding is in the eating!"

CHAPTER 1

Many thousands of years ago, by the bank of the Yamunā River, on a shallow inlet where the waters slowed and widened into a haven for warm-water fish, lay an old fishing village named Kalpi. Everyone had always called it Dāśa-grāma, Fisher Village, and the simplicity of its inhabitants made its simple name appropriate.

The village had a leader, who called himself Dāśa-rāja, the fisher king. He insisted that his wife be addressed as Dāśa-rājñī, the fisher queen. Being naturally humble, she tolerated rather than enjoyed this name.

With a strong will, and a secret supply of gold coins, Dāśa-rāja ruled the village. Within his humble means (he would not spend his gold coins), he tried to dress, walk, and speak like a king. He even tried to move his weather-beaten head and leathery hands with royal dignity. His wife, indifferent to her husband's royal pretensions, thought of her family's health and comfort, and little else.

This fishing folk lived in cottages woven of thick straw, with palm thatch roofs, each dwelling fronted by an earthen patio, smooth as glass, and swept morning and evening with straw brooms. The inhabitants drew fresh water from the river, and had never dug a well.

Sitting in their huts, or in the deep shade of mango and banyan trees, villagers sharpened knives and mended nets. Others tended vegetable gardens, cut fish and fruit, cooked and nursed. Fishers filled the inlet in boats and rafts.

Broken old boats leaned against coconut and banana trees. Barking dogs completed the landscape. The villagers communicated primarily by shouting, even to those near them. The stench of dead fish scented the air.

The king and queen of Dāśa Village had a very lovely daughter, Satya-vatī, their only child. She absolutely refused to be called fisher princess. Ironically, her extraordinary beauty and poise made her the only resident of that village for whom a royal name would not seem absurd to a visitor. Her sixteenth birthday had come and gone. The seventeenth approached. Each passing day deepened her disappointment with life. She did not like to fish, nor harm any other creature. The stench of dead fish sickened her. So, she served her parents by ferrying travelers across the river for a small fee. Her father always claimed to need money. Satya knew he hoarded his gold against future troubles, which always remained undefined.

As a young girl, she spent her days on the river. Around a sharp bend, she had found a small, abandoned island, and made it her secret, magic place. Here, as a child, she ate sweet, wild fruits and dreamed of visiting Śukti-matī, the great capital of her country, Cedi. There, she would meet the royal family, and dance at royal balls.

One day, years ago, when she was eight years old, her life had suddenly changed. Across the river was a village of elderly brāhmaṇa sages. They were kind but never mixed with the fishing folk. As a young girl, Satya-vatī brought passengers to and from the village, but never tarried there. The sages were far above her in the social order. She did sometimes sense that the sages carefully watched her, but she dismissed her thought as foolish.

Then one day, after taking visitors to the brāhmaṇa village, two sages approached her, and actually said that they wished to visit her village. This startled her. Sages never visited the fishing folk, though the fishers, hoping for material blessings, sometimes sent small gifts to the sages with those crossing the river.

Young Satya nervously bowed to the two sages and welcomed them into her small craft. As they crossed the river, the sages spoke to her kindly, trying to make her feel at ease. Indeed, anyone could see how nervous she was.

Upon arriving, she took them to her parents' hut and waited outside. She heard the sages speaking to her parents. She could not make out their words. The talk was short. The brāhmaṇas came out. She was to take them back to their village. They set off. She was too shy to study their faces for clues. Halfway across the river, a sage said, "Dear girl, you will come several times a week to study with us. Your parents agreed. You will begin tomorrow."

After the first wave of incredulity, Satya was too happy to speak or even to smile. Letting go of her rudder for just a moment, she clasped her hands and bowed to the sages. She had longed to study, to know the wide world, the histories of heroic kings, the wisdom of the hallowed Veda. None of that was possible at home. She could not imagine why the sages had chosen her, and dared not ask. She concluded that her dear Yamunā, the river goddess, had given her this blessing.

The next day her education began. The young girl was ecstatic, for her brilliant mind received nourishment at last. She brought little gifts for the sages — milk sweets and fruit baskets, and helped them with their chores. They sat with her under the shade of ancient mango trees, near the shore where the Yamunā's waters lapped the silver sand.

She knew her father was not pleased with her studies, but he dared not oppose the sages. They were holy. They had powers. At first, Satya-vatī tried to share with her parents the knowledge that so inspired her. But they were always busy or bored, till one day, her father chastised her, shouting that she should not try to be better than her parents in *anything*. It was not her place to instruct them.

Satya did not reply, but his words wounded her. She could not see him the same after that, though she did not betray her change of heart.

Her heart and mind no longer dwelled in the fishing village. She dreamed of visiting the great nations she had learned of from the sages — the Kurus, Yadus, and Pañcālas. Most of all Satya-vatī yearned to visit Śukti-matī, Pearl River, the great capital of her own Cedi nation. Studies on contemporary political events fascinated her, which was quite unusual for a member of the humble fishing community of Kalpi.

In the sand, the sages drew maps of Cedi and nearby kingdoms, and their glorious capitals, and told her the distance to each. Soon Satya could draw the maps herself, with great capitals like Hastinā-pura, Kāmpilya, and Mathurā, and her own Śukti-matī.

Most thrilling was a description of Cedi's king, *her king*, great Vasu, who had risen to the status of *king of kings*, and flew about the world in a crystal airship given to him by the Deva lord, Indra. Satya-vatī never tired of hearing about King Vasu, and his lovely, brilliant wife, Queen Girikā.

As her studies progressed, Satya gave up the crude speech of the fishing village. She now spoke with the elegant diction of her learned gurus. But her parents resented and mistrusted her fine speech. To avoid endless quarrels, she spoke crudely in the fishing village, and increasingly yearned to escape its confines.

For eight years, Satya-vatī eagerly studied, continuing to contribute to the family economy by ferrying travelers across the river for an hour or two each day.

By now, Satya spoke like a most learned child of sages. She knew well the exploits of current and past kings, the history of countries with their alliances, victories, and defeats. She mastered geography, logic, political science, and current affairs. She now debated and discoursed on these topics, under the proud, watchful eyes of her teachers.

But all this she concealed from her parents and the other fishing folk. Her father continued to resent his daughter knowing more than her father about anything, and the simple villagers felt obliged to share his view. Her mother echoed her husband's views, though without real conviction.

As Satya blossomed into a strikingly beautiful young lady, her parents found a new cause of dissatisfaction with her. She refused to choose a husband among the fisher boys.

One day, Satya's parents came to her as she sat by the river, facing the dawn, quietly reciting her lessons. She braced herself for the predictable speech.

"Young lady," her mother began, "our life is one of joy and grief."

Satya could not stand to hear this again.

"My love," her mother sighed, "the village talks about you. If you don't marry soon, what will everyone say? You are such a beauty; the best boys in the village would do anything to win your hand. Handsome boys."

"But they're not good enough for you," her father grumbled. "No, you're too good for all of them."

"Father, *please*." Satya tried to calm him, but it never worked.

"Handsome boys, strong boys." Dāśa-rāja was nearly shouting. "But not good enough for you."

His wife, the fisher queen, sighed. "Why won't you do your duty?"

Satya was desperate to escape. "How many times will we talk about this? I like the boys, but as brothers! I won't marry them. I wouldn't be happy."

"But why?" her father insisted. "You tell me why."

"You know why." She raised her own voice. "I'm sorry, I really am. But I will not spend the rest of my life here."

"You're ashamed of your own people who raised and loved you!" her mother cried.

"I'm not ashamed! I'm *different*!" Satya cried. "You know I am. I don't fit here."

Her parents eyed each other. Her father fell to muttering. Her mother made a grieving sound. Satya-vatī bowed to them, and ran to a secluded mango grove, weeping in frustration beneath the leafy trees.

Satya *was* different, and whenever she said it, her parents had no reply. In her earliest childhood games, she was not a fisher girl, but a princess in a royal court. As years passed, her dreams grew more real. She married a mighty young king, inspiring him to fight evil and protect the innocent. She gave bountiful charity to all in need. She sat on a jeweled throne and granted the petitions of loyal subjects.

Her parents knew of her fantasies, and dismissed them as innocent games. But to Satya, this world of dreams was far more real than the oppressive monotony of a small fishing village. Indeed, when she thought of spending all her life here, she could hardly breathe. Her parents' plea to marry horrified her, for marriage in the village would trap her for the rest of her life.

But today was a new day, and time for her lessons across the river. She ran to the sandy shore and gazed at the river in the soft early light. If only she could float away to another world. The idea thrilled and pained her. If she left the village, she would betray her people. If she stayed, she would betray herself.

Across the wide and sacred Yamunā, fragrant smoke rose from the offering fires of the learned brāhmaṇas. She was eager to see the elderly sages she adored, and who adored her no less. She might not reach another world today, but she would escape for a while!

She startled her mother with eager words. "Please give me sweets. I'm crossing to the brāhmaṇa village. I must bring a gift." Satya looked across the river and saw the wisps of curling smoke from sacred fires. Soon the sages would be telling stories. She wanted to cross the river now.

"Why go there now?" Her father shook his weather-beaten head, and lifted his leathery hands for emphasis. "We have work to do. You could mend nets. You've learned enough. More than you need."

Satya-vatī shook her head and smiled. She raised her hands and said, "Father, the Veda says we must serve the wise. You've always taught that. I don't only study, I help the elderly sages. That is our duty, and our whole family receives blessings from that service. The Veda says that!"

"What do I know of Veda? I know we have our work to do," her father said brusquely, "For now, the sages across the river are doing just fine. We have our own work to do, and my daughter should be here helping her parents."

"But the sages need our care," Satya insisted. "They are all so elderly and have no families to look after them. I must go."

Dāśa-rāja did not reply. Satya kept silent. Her father didn't need her help if he would only spend a fraction of the gold coins he hoarded.

"All right," her mother said. "We're tired of fighting with you. Cross the river if you like. You're a young lady now. May the Devas protect you."

"Yes, the Devas and mighty King Vasu!" Satya cried. "He loves his people and we love him. Remember how he and Queen Girikā visited Kalpi when I was small? He was so handsome and kind. Why didn't he come back? Mother, will we ever see King Vasu again? Will he return?"

"Stop dreaming, young girl." Her mother put down her needles. "The great King Vasu will not return to a poor, little fishing village."

"Then why don't we go to the capital, Śukti-matī? It's not so far."

"My dear girl, the capital is farther than you think, and we will not go. We struggle daily to put food in your mouth, and you think we can sail off to a big city?"

"But will I ever see the king again?"

"Your father is a king, and you see him every day. If only you would listen to him!"

"Oh, Mother! I would love to visit the great capital of Cedi! They say His Majesty and beautiful Queen Girikā live in a jeweled palace with the loveliest gardens."

"Oh, how you dream, young lady. We would all get lost in Pearl River. And people there would laugh at us. We are plain folk, and capital folk are rich and fancy. No, let us stay here and do our duty. That pleases the Devas."

"Well, I'm going to see the brāhmaṇas now," Satya said.

Her father grumbled. Her mother sighed and said, "All right, dearest, if you must. Take sweets from the shelf. Beg the sages to bless our family and our village and the souls of the departed."

"Of course, Mother." Satya-vatī grabbed the sweets and turned to leave, when her father blurted out, "Wait a moment young lady!"

He closed his eyes as he always did when trying to decide a difficult issue. He opened his eyes. "There's another thing. I hesitated to tell you, but I will now. It may not be safe to visit the brāhmaṇas. You may have to stop your study."

Satya-vatī opened her eyes wide. "Not safe? What are you saying?"

"I mean your mother and I heard stories. We didn't want to scare you. But we've been hearing stories like we never heard before. Wild beasts, demon-possessed, attack and kill sages in the deep forest."

"It's too horrible to repeat!" the fisher queen said. "Cruel, evil beasts! Demon-possessed. The beasts go straight for the brāhmaṇas."

"As if they know what they're doing!" the fisher king said.

"Who told you that?" Satya demanded, deeply alarmed.

"It was a traveler; I don't remember his name."

"Where did this happen?"

"It was in several kingdoms," her father said. "I can't remember the names. But what the man told us was sickening. And he knew. And now, they say it's coming closer!"

"That is awful, if it's true," Satya said, doubting the story. Her father told many stories.

"Of course it's true!" her father shouted.

"But why didn't you tell me before?" Satya said.

"Because it was far from here," her father said. "Faraway kingdoms. We didn't want to frighten you."

"Yes!" Her mother added, "Don't talk about trouble and trouble won't find you. I learned that from my parents."

"But it's coming," her father said. "Oh yes, it's coming."

Satya-vatī doubted these stories. Her parents always told her stories of evil spirits that steal bad children. Her mother was very superstitious, and recited many folk spells to ward off all manner of evil and danger. Satya knew this was quite normal among the fisher folk. As a child, she had believed it all. As a young lady, she tolerated it as the typical superstitions of simple people.

Now, Satya just wanted to calm her parents and get away to her boat. "I see. I understand your concern. But surely King Vasu will protect his own land of Cedi. Brāhmaṇas are safe in Cedi, as long as King Vasu rules."

The fisher king scowled. "Yes, we hope the king does his duty, but…"

She was desperate to change the subject. "Oh, how I long to go to the capital, to see our king."

"Oh, Satya!" her mother cried. "Just stay here where you're safe, though I do thank the Devas that mighty King Vasu protects all his people."

Seeing her father about to speak again, Satya-vatī hurried off. Could the stories be true? King Vasu possessed a heavily armed crystal craft that moved at his will. If dark forces had come to Earth and were attacking the sages, could the king stop them? Were any of them safe?

CHAPTER 2

Satya-vatī jumped into to her boat, struggling to put the terrible stories out of her mind. Her parents had no proof of the atrocities.

As the newborn sun flashed in the forest and sparkled on the river, Satya-vatī pushed off into the river. Still troubled by what she heard, she lay on her back and breathed deeply, letting the boat drift where it would. Her large eyes gazed at the rich blue sky and whitening clouds.

After minutes of a troubled reverie, she sat up briskly, gripped the stern oar with strong, young hands, and steered the craft over rippling waters to the far bank. A smile lit her face as she waved to the old sages, busy with ablutions at water's edge. They cried out to her, accenting the last syllable: "Satya-va-tee! Satya-va-tee!"

Satya jumped from her boat and pulled it onto the soft, silver bank. Her fine young figure complemented the startling beauty of her face, with its arresting eyes, graceful nose, soft, shapely lips, and teeth white as jasmine buds.

She bowed to the sages, touching her curling, silken hair to the sand. She stood up, arched her back, straightened her dress, and brushed sand from her hair, as the sages happily welcomed her into their midst. They loved her from her childhood, and she loved them. To think of these pure souls in danger from unnatural beasts sent a chill up her spine. But she would not let her parents frighten her into compliance with their wishes for her life.

She strolled about, greeting the elderly sages, whom she called *grandfather*, happily placing sweets in their aged hands. They taught her all she knew of the world beyond her village. And she had served them faithfully.

Her eyes glimpsed a *young* sage. He was her age, or a bit older. Who was he? Only older sages came to this āśrama. Curiosity seized her.

The youth, with his high, handsome forehead, sat pensively near the river. His smooth, dark hair fell gently on his bare shoulders. He meditated with half-closed eyes.

Satya wandered in his direction, never moving straight toward him, but walking this way and that, stopping to examine a flower, turning to exchange a word with an elderly sage, turning again as if to see if the river was still there, but steadily closing the distance between her and the young sage.

She stopped twenty yards to his right, as he sat facing the river. She would come no closer. Trying to appear indifferent, looking at other things, Satya slowly brought him within her sight.

"He's so different from the fishing boys," she thought with a flutter. "He's more like me. But how is he like me? What could I possibly mean?"

Lost in these musings, she forgot her caution and actually stared at the young sage. Meditating with half-open eyes, as ancient texts prescribe, he noticed her. He met her eyes with his piercing and equally innocent gaze. Startled, Satya-vatī quickly turned away, but she could not avoid the blush that spread over her cheeks.

Normally graceful, Satya awkwardly retreated, almost tripping as she feigned a calm continuation of her walk. He called out to her, "Please! Wait!"

Eyes glued to her feet, she turned back, joined her hands in respect, and said, "Yes, brāhmaṇa, how may I serve you?"

He stood and came her way. She bowed her head and he bowed his in return. Why did he do that? She bowed again, fearing her hot face was red. He smiled. She knew he knew her thoughts.

In a clear voice, fearless in its innocence, he asked, "May I speak to you, good maiden?"

"If that is your wish, brāhmaṇa," she replied. She sat with him on soft grass by the river. He faced her. She faced the river.

"Are you Satya-vatī?" he asked.

"Yes, sage." She assumed he learned her name from the older sages.

"You live nearby, I believe?"

"Yes," she said, both flattered and sad. He must know she was a fisher's daughter. Never before had Satya felt ashamed of her own family. She rebuked herself. Though she could not accept her life in a fishing village, she loved her family and people, as they loved her. It seemed proper that a river separated the fishers from brāhmaṇas who lived in a superior world.

But now, meeting this young sage, the first noble youth she ever met, irrepressible shame filled her heart. A painful truth afflicted her: she was low, and this handsome boy was high. To this was added the greater shame of betraying the very people who loved and raised her.

All these thoughts assaulted her in an instant. She struggled to mask her turmoil with a calm appearance. "If I may ask, sage, what is your name?"

"I am Parā-śara."

Satya-vatī, who had been steadily staring at the ground, now looked up in surprise. "You are Parā-śara? Oh, but that must be a name shared by brāhmaṇas. I assume you are not the ancient sage Parā-śara."

He smiled. "Yes, I am that Parā-śara."

How could this youth be the legendary brāhmaṇa she had heard of since childhood? Curiosity overcame her and the words flew from her lips. "But how can you be so young? Is it by yoga power?"

He smiled with kind amusement and nodded. His kindness emboldened her. She continued, "When I was small, the brāhmaṇas told me that long ago you made a mighty offering into sacred fire and destroyed the Rakṣas who threatened the world. I loved that story."

He smiled and nodded. "Your martial spirit pleases me, though it does not surprise me."

What could he mean? How could he know her? His relaxed manner gave her confidence to ask more questions. She decided to ask him whether savage beasts were really attacking brāhmaṇas in far-off lands. But as she was gathering courage to ask, she heard a far shout and paddle splash. She turned to look. Oh no! Her father, for spite or caprice, had sent a fisher boy to call her back home.

Parā-śara must not see her with that boy, a boy who wanted to marry her. If she didn't go now, her father would send more boys, the whole village if necessary.

She begged the sage's forgiveness and declared she must leave at once. He smiled and spoke the words she longed to hear,

"Will you please come again tomorrow?"

"If you wish, sage," replied Satya-vatī, trying to look calm.

"I do wish it. Thank you. And I must beg you, do not tell anyone who I am. The motive for secrecy will become clear in time."

"Of course," she said, " but don't all these sages know you?"

"They know me only as a young brāhmaṇa. I came here just to see you. No one else."

"I assure you," she said with a blush impossible to hide, "I will keep your secret."

She bowed, confused and giddy. The fishing boat came near. She dashed to her own boat, bowing her head to the sages as she ran, begging them to forgive her hasty departure, and ignoring the calls of the fisher boy. She rowed strongly back so he could not catch her. With every stroke, the sage's words echoed in her mind: "I came just to see you. No one else." What did he think of her? Would he take her away to a new life? But as she neared her village, other more troubling thoughts arose.

Flattering as it was, *why* did he come to see her? Why *her*? Parā-śara was an enlightened sage. He must know the truth about the animal attacks. She would ask him tomorrow, and if he knew *anything* about it, she would immediately send the news to her own dear king, Vasu. No! She would go to Śukti-matī and personally bring him the information!

But if Parā-śara's sudden appearance was related to the animal attacks, could her own dear sages be in danger? She gasped at the thought. She suspected that something extraordinary was happening in the world, and she was somehow involved!

Why had the brāhmaṇas chosen her as their student? As an eight-year-old girl, she had attributed this blessing to dear Yamunā. She still believed this, but the brāhmaṇas themselves must have had some reason. She had never asked, but now it struck her as exceedingly unusual. And Parā-śara! Could all these facts be related?

Lost in thought, she forgot where she was till her boat bumped into the little village dock.

CHAPTER 3

Satya-vatī now had to contend with her father. She knew what he would say. And he said it: "You stayed too long! We are simple people. We raised you. You must help us. You cannot spend all day with the brāhmaṇas."

"I always do my work," Satya said with a scowl.

"All right, don't get angry with me." Her father shook his head and walked away. The next day, eager to see Parā-śara, she decided to return at dawn to the brāhmaṇa village.

"Why do you go now, so early?" her father grumbled.

"A sage asked for my help. I gave my word."

"What sage?" her father demanded.

"I forgot his name. He has one of those typical brāhmaṇa names like Bhārgava or Gautama."

"Satya!" cried her mother. "Respect the sages and remember their names, or the Devas will punish you."

"I will," Satya promised. Her father put a big, leathery hand on her shoulder and said, "The Devas created people different, high and low. We are not meant to be with brāhmaṇas. Listen to me. Enough is enough. I don't approve of more trips across the river."

"Father!" Satya cried. "I like the sages and they like me. They never tell me not to come. I'd rather die than be trapped here all my life!"

Shocking herself, as well as her parents, with these bold words, Satya ran before they could reply, jumped into her boat, and pushed off before they could stop her. She was truly eager to see the sages. But her thoughts of one young sage in particular drove her forward.

On the opposite shore, she greeted the elderly brāhmaṇas, but did not see Parā-śara. Where was he? She told the brāhmaṇas she would bring them kindling from the forest and ran to look for Parā-śara.

She found him in the woods seated alone. Both their faces brightened on meeting. With a gracious gesture, he invited her to sit by him. She sat gratefully at a respectful distance and bowed her head.

"I admire your courage in coming here," he said. "I expected that from you."

"Thank you," she replied, intrigued by his words. Why did he expect her to be courageous? She waited, too shy to ask. He spoke again in a soft voice. "I came to you because the world is in danger, and you must help to protect it."

He astonished her. What did he mean? Still, her heart swelled at his inscrutable faith in her.

"Brāhmaṇa," she said, "we see no great threat to our world. I have heard that terrible beasts have attacked brāhmaṇas in faraway lands. I fear my father exaggerates, based on rumors. If what he says is true, and I seek your guidance here, then I grieve for those poor sages more than I can say. But, generally, goodness fills our world. Peace and prosperity reign. Here in Cedi, we have a powerful king, Vasu, who protects us all. Indeed, he is king of kings and protects many lands."

Parā-śara nodded. "All you say is true. This world has recently lived a golden age of virtue, peace, and prosperity. But I say truly, Satya-vatī, danger stalks your world. And that danger is related to the stories, which are true, of attacks on sages."

"Oh God!" Satya cried. "Please, tell me what is happening."

Parā-śara breathed deeply, and looked toward heaven. Then he faced Satya and said, "The dangers we face today began far from this world. A fierce war broke out between two cosmic forces — the Devas, who protect the three worlds (the upper, middle and lower worlds), and the Asuras, who would enslave the worlds for their pleasure."

"Parā-śara," she said, "everyone heard of that war, but we know so little about it, only that the Devas bravely defeated the Asuras and saved the three worlds."

"That is almost correct, Satya-vatī. With Viṣṇu's help, the Devas did defeat the marauding Asuras in an epic *battle*. But people on Earth do not know that the *war itself* did not end."

"What are you saying?" Satya asked.

"Listen with full attention to my words. You will see all that I describe as if you were there."

With a gasp of excited anticipation, Satya sat quickly and firmly in a perfect meditation posture. Since childhood she had studied and imitated sages and yogīs, mastering their postures, and naturally imbibing their gravity and powers of concentration. She hid this power from her simple parents. Now she summoned it.

Parā-śara's eyes glowed with approval as he watched her. "So that you understand what we face, and what we must do, I will take you back in time."

CHAPTER 4

At Parā-śara's behest, Satya entered into deep meditation. As he spoke, Satya strained to his every word, and she began to see all he described as if she were there.

On the wings of his words, she gazed in wonder at Tri-kūṭa, the fabled three-peaked mountain that rose from the great milk-white sea to unfathomed heights. Parā-śara revealed to her the celestial realm!

Satya-vatī flew at mind-speed into Tri-kūṭa's verdant valleys. She waved to its playful, colorful creatures even though they could not see her. She sailed over forests ablaze with flowers and fruits she had never seen before. Singing, soaring birds swelled the heavens with song. Satya glided over crystalline rivers and lakes with banks of soft, jeweled sand. Finally, she reached the Great White Sea, whose milky waves, lapping the beach, transformed sand into emeralds.

This was the Deva realm! Indeed, there on that shining, dark-green beach, the Devas, rulers of the three worlds, were camped. But as Satya drew near, her euphoria turned to alarm. Danger stalked. The Milk Sea's dancing waves grew wild, crashing with fury on darkening shores. Parā-śara had led her not to a heavenly pleasure ground but to a war ground. Deva armies gathered below. Chilling winds made Satya shiver.

She descended into the bustling, bright-flagged war camp of the Devas, pulsing with latent battle. Parā-śara brought her into the finest tent, where lovely Śacī, Indra's consort, queen of heaven, gazed into a floating jeweled mirror at her unaging face. She lifted a finger to her soft cheek, studied the big reflected eyes, and trembled with fear.

Śacī gazed upon her husband, Indra, the Deva king, who lay resting on sheets softer and whiter than any earthly cloth. Even in rest, Indra breathed power. Śacī watched her sleeping mate, with his fine gold locks and flawless face. But dread, not joy, sculpted her features.

The commotion of a rapidly approaching chariot flying white banners, drawn by two mighty horses, purple and white, drew Satya's attention. Into the tent rushed an imposing celestial prince. From all she had learned, Satya recognized him at once. It was the handsome Deva Vāyu, guardian of the celestial northwest. Indra's nephew Yama, lord of the celestial south who judges the dead, came after him. With bows to Śacī, they went to Indra's bedside and he instantly awoke.

"It is war!" they cried. "Asuras march against us."

Instantly focused, Indra rose. Placing a golden helmet over his golden hair, he asked, "Are you absolutely sure?"

"Listen!" Vāyu said. "The wind carries their war cries."

Indra heard and fixed his armor. Śacī sighed. She knew it would come to this. Looking out from the jeweled tent, she saw Devas frantically readying for battle. Vāyu and Yama left to rejoin their troops, allowing the couple some privacy. Indra turned to her and said, "Śacī, are you all right?"

"Me? Yes, of course."

He took her in his arms and said, "This must be difficult for you."

"I worry about you, Indra. They chose to fight you." Śacī closed her eyes in fear. "They chose..."

"If it was me alone they came to fight, I could walk away for your sake, for the sake of peace. But they attack the Law. They attack Dharma, and thereby threaten the three worlds."

"I know," Śacī said. "I grew up with them. I knew when I married you it would come to this. After all, unlike you, I was not born to Devas. I am an Asura's daughter."

"I love you," Indra insisted. "I don't care about your birth."

"But my father..." she said.

"Yes, your father, Pulomā, has proved to be..."

"One of the worst Asuras, I know," Śacī said, downcast. "And his two brothers, my uncles Vṛṣa-parva, king of the Asuras, and Vipra-citti, the most powerful Asura. That was my family. Yet their mother, Danu, my grandmother, is a Devī, a goddess like your mother, Aditi. If only my father and all the Asuras would join the Devas. They could rule the worlds together. There would be peace at last."

Indra sat down and pulled Śacī onto his lap. He stroked her shining hair and whispered, "I'm sorry, Śacī, but you know what I must do today."

"I know. But they will try to kill you, and they have terrible powers."

"What has their guru Śukra taught them now?" Indra asked.

"I don't know. They don't confide in me. They see how much I love you."

"As I love you. But the Asuras do not care for the warrior code. The Law, Dharma, means nothing to them. If we press them, they may resort to the Dark Magic."

"What will you do, Indra?"

"Śacī, what can we do? We must turn to the Avatāra, Viṣṇu. Only Viṣṇu can save us then."

"But will the Avatāra come?"

"Let us hope so," Indra said.

Indra held Śacī tight. They heard quick steps. Vāyu and Yama returned with the young twin Aśvins, most handsome of Devas. Śacī stood with Indra to receive the Deva generals.

"Ready?" Indra asked.

"Yes!" Vāyu smiled. "I look forward to the battle."

"I do not," Yama said. "You know I will fight. Still, the Asuras are half-brothers, uncles, nephews, cousins. I do not welcome their deaths."

"I am sworn to defend the Law," Indra said, "and they are sworn to destroy it. We vow to defend the world, and our Asura family vows to enslave it."

"If only we could persuade them," Yama said.

Indra smiled. "Kindness clouds your mind. They will live and die as Asuras. And if one of them chose peace, the others would kill him."

"But someday," Yama said, "the worlds must unite. We must strive for peace."

Vāyu laughed. "Yama! You of all Devas dream of peace in this world, you who judge and punish the wicked! Surely by now your job has made you cynical. Do you believe that all souls will someday be good?"

"Someday all souls will return to their pure nature," Yama insisted.

"Yes, and that is fine talk," Indra said, "but today's event is war. The Asuras will soon attack."

"May Viṣṇu be with us," Śacī said.

"I pray," Indra said, "that we will not trouble him today."

Śacī and other Devī goddesses left their tents and rose into the sky in celestial aircrafts to watch the battle from a safe distance. Below on the emerald shore of the Great White Ocean, proud banners whipped in the wind. Celestial horns and drums resounded.

From just over the horizon, a terrible clamor burst forth, rending sky and mind. Vast Asura legions poured into the plain between sea and mountain. Deva shouts thundered as raging armies rushed against each other, hurling oaths and weapons.

By Law, by Dharma, infantry fought infantry, cavalry attacked cavalry, chariots battled chariots. Weapons clashed with equal weapons in terrifying tests of skill and courage. In a fair fight, Devas led by Indra pushed back Asuras.

Indra and Vāyu led the Devas. Yama fought with striking valor. Śacī watched anxiously as the young twin Aśvins challenged her father's brother, the Asura king, Vṛṣa-parva. Vāyu attacked Śacī's father, Pulomā. Śacī closed her eyes in fear. When she opened them, she saw her father and uncle alive, though struggling.

When desperate Asura commanders converged on Indra, Śacī shuddered. But Indra rose above them, cutting Asura weapons to pieces before they left his enemy's hand.

She saw her husband lift his dreaded Vajra thunderbolt. She saw her father move toward Indra. Śacī prayed, "Let it not be." Indra looked up at her, and moved away from her father. Śacī sank down on her seat and wept. If only the fight would end now.

When Deva victory seemed certain, the Asuras vanished into the air. Devas shouted, "Dark Magic! Beware the Dark Magic!"

It was not long in coming. A huge stone mountain flashed into the sky above the Devas, who looked up in horror. "Cowards!" Indra cried at the Asuras. "Fight like warriors. Do not hide behind a coward's sorcery. Dharma forbids Dark Magic. Fight fairly! Damn your Asura tricks!"

Śacī screamed for Indra and his army to flee as the hovering Asura mountain exploded into flames. Fiery trees and razor-sharp stones rained down, shredding the Deva army. Giant serpents and scorpions rushed on them. Giant lions, tigers, boars, and elephants ravaged them.

Naked, spike-wielding demonesses and cannibal hordes attacked, screaming, "Slice the Devas! Pierce them!" In the wind-blasted sky, roaring clouds gushed live coals and lightning. Floods of gale-driven fire razed heaven's troops. Pitched and flung by fierce wind, the sea hurtled past its shore, unleashing swirling terror. Vāyu cried out, for he could not control his own wind-domain. Indra cursed, for rain and lightning did not obey him.

Proud Indra would not appeal for Viṣṇu's help. He fought on, but the Dark Magic steadily overcame his legions. Finally, Vāyu, Yama, and the Aśvins looked over the White Sea to White Island, Viṣṇu's abode. They pleaded and demanded that Indra beg Viṣṇu to come.

"Forget the glory, Indra! Call him now!"

Still, Indra hesitated, unable to accept that he could not defend the world from the Asuras. Again, the Devas urged him, "Please, Indra, you must invoke Viṣṇu. We can't hold out."

When Indra again hesitated, Deva forces sank into despair and terror. Even Indra now looked across the White Sea to White Island, the mystic abode of Viṣṇu. Indra and his Devas could not contend with the Dark Magic.

Mighty, lion-mounted Kāla-nemi, a ferocious Asura, exploited the confusion and fell on the Devas with cruel, bow-shot missiles. The harsh twang of his infamous bow so unnerved the Devas that some dropped their weapons, fell to their knees, and begged him to spare their lives. Others fled madly before his onslaught. If a Deva dared stand and fight Kāla-nemi, his leader Vipra-citti rushed to his support, and they both killed the Deva. Vipra-citti would then raise arms with Kāla-nemi, and they roared in jubilation. When Kāla-nemi so terrified some Devas that they dropped their weapons and shields, or fell from their chariots, Kāla-nemi ridiculed them and did not kill them.

Seeing this, Indra now fixed his desperate mind on Avatāra Viṣṇu. The Devas all followed him. The Asuras felt the force of this meditation. Gazing respectively in hope and dread toward the glowing White Island, Devas and Asuras all saw the luminous Avatāra rise above his island on the back of his deadly eagle, Garuḍa, quickly cross the Great White Sea, and descend toward the battlefield.

As Viṣṇu approached, all the Dark Magic vanished. Gone was the killing mountain, gone the fires, animals, snakes, and naked demonesses. The sea calmed. Through a threatening sky, Viṣṇu Avatāra came near.

Hovering above the war field, he extended one hand to the Devas, one to the Asuras, speaking peace, urging both sides to accept the just Law, Dharma, that defends all who defend it. The Devas bowed their heads to Viṣṇu, laying down their weapons. But some Asuras defiantly brandished their weapons, shouting vulgar threats against Viṣṇu.

Kāla-nemi hated the Avatāra. Riding his giant lion, not waiting for his commander's order, he rushed in rage at Viṣṇu, whirled his razor spear, and, with a scream, sped it at blinding speed toward the Avatāra, who still extended an open hand to the Asuras. With that very hand, Viṣṇu seized the spear and hurled it back with such force that it burst through Kāla-nemi and his lion mount and buried itself in the emerald shore. For one moment, Kāla-nemi stared with shock, fear, and rage at the Avatāra, then fell dead on that shore.

Asuras, Devas, and their wives all watched transfixed. Vipra-citti tried to rally Asura warriors to fight the Avatāra and avenge Kāla-nemi. Two deadly Asuras, Mālī and Su-mālī, furiously charged the Avatāra, who calmly raised his hand. Atop his skyward index finger, a blazing whirling disc appeared. As the two Asuras roared and aimed weapons, the disc raced toward them with heart-stopping speed, sliced off their heads, hovered eerily in the air for a moment, and then returned to Viṣṇu's finger.

Vipra-citti gripped his weapons but did not raise them, and Viṣṇu did not attack him. But Asura Mālya-vān, in blind fury, rushed Viṣṇu with a spiked club and lost his head to the blazing disc. No other Asura came forward, though Vipra-citti uttered silent oaths. Viṣṇu nodded to the Devas and to those Asuras who did not attack him. Having stopped the Dark Magic, he flew from the battlefield, back to his White Island.

The Asuras stared at one another in confusion. Vipra-citti praised, promised, and rebuked them till they again attacked the Devas. But Indra rallied the Devas, who in fair combat shattered the Asura legions. Vāyu, Indra, and other Devas slew the relentless Asuras as lions slay deer.

Seeing the Asuras' imminent extinction, the revered sage Nārada flew to the battlefield and cried out: "Devas! Victory is yours. Avatāra Viṣṇu favored you, for you follow Dharma. He preserved your just rule of the three worlds. You flourish, Devas! Now, end this fighting!"

CARTOGRAPHY OF THE MAHĀ-BHĀRATA

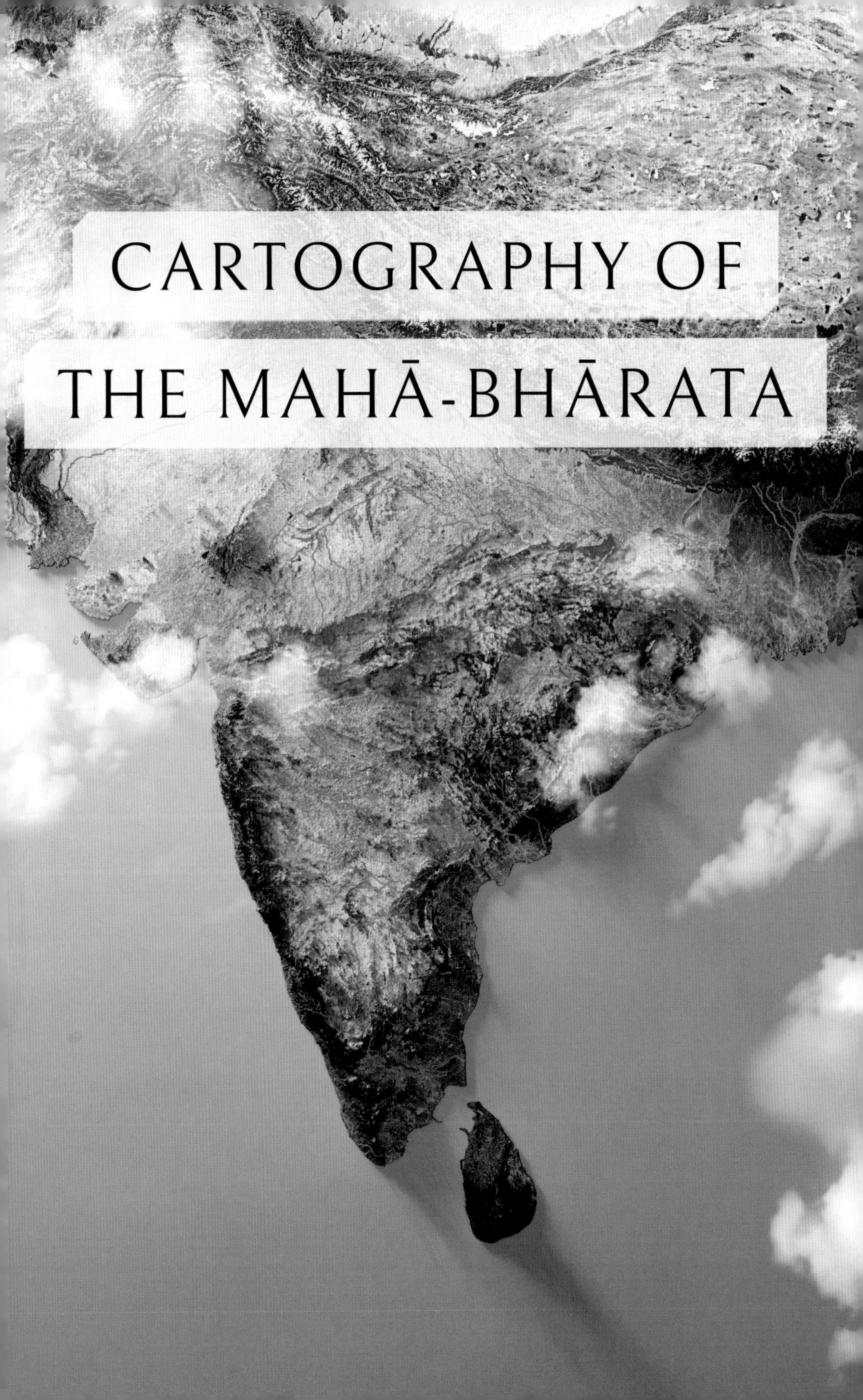

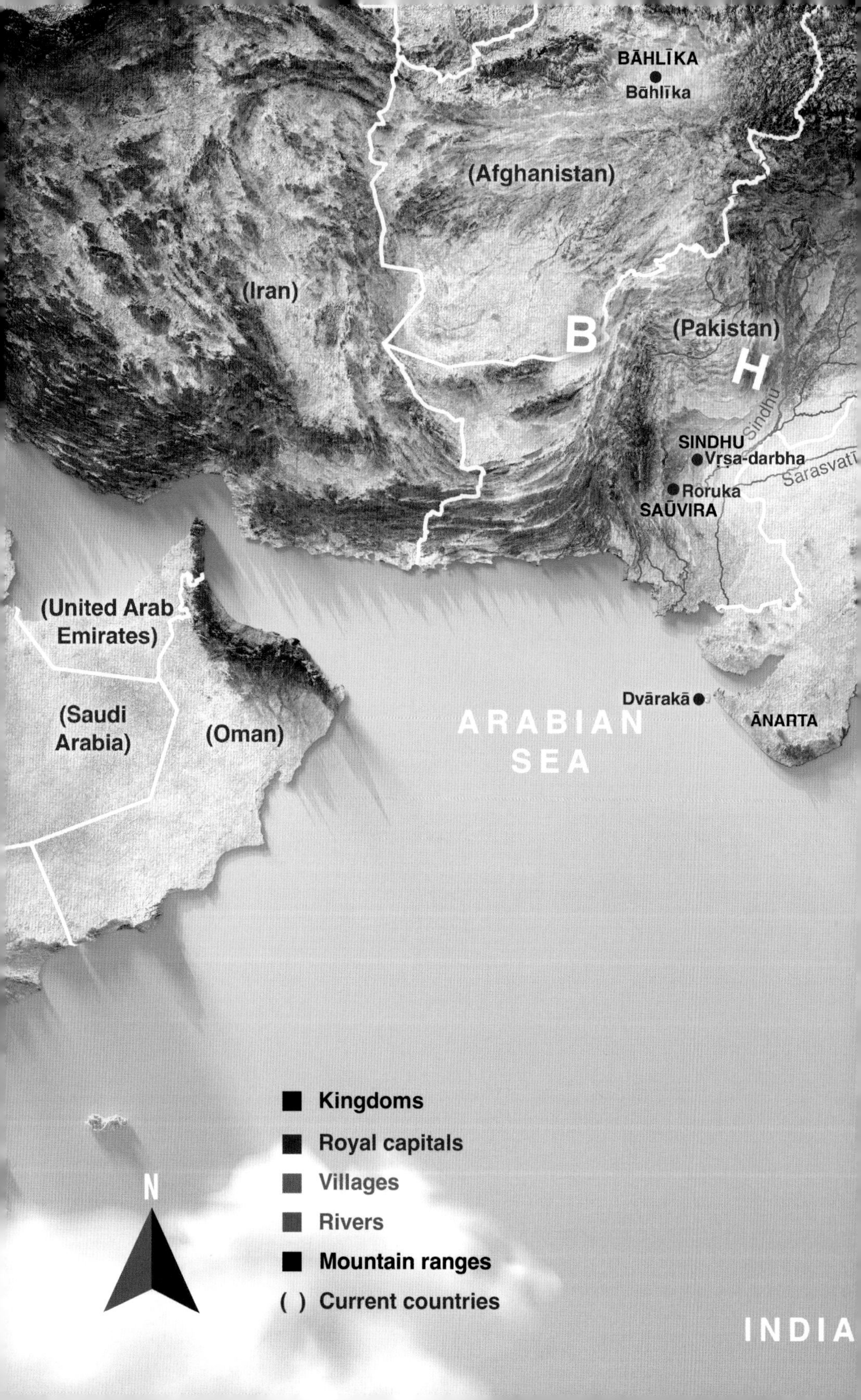
BĀHLĪKA
Bāhlīka
(Afghanistan)
(Iran)
B
(Pakistan)
H
Sindhu
SINDHU
Vṛṣa-darbha
Sarasvatī
Roruka
SAŪVIRA
(United Arab Emirates)
(Saudi Arabia)
(Oman)
Dvārakā
ĀNARTA
ARABIAN SEA
Kingdoms
Royal capitals
Villages
Rivers
Mountain ranges
( ) Current countries
N
INDIA

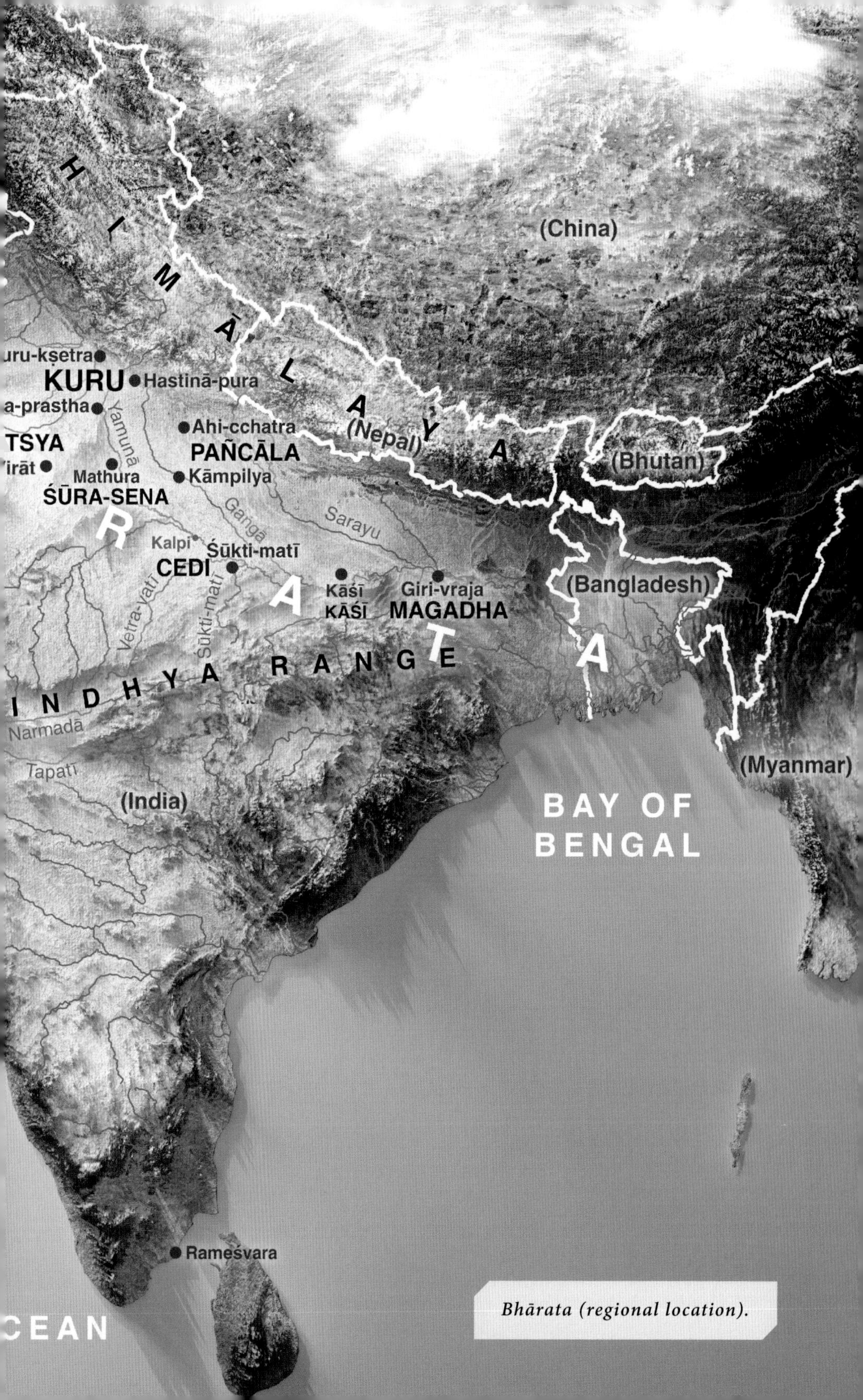

Bhārata (regional location).

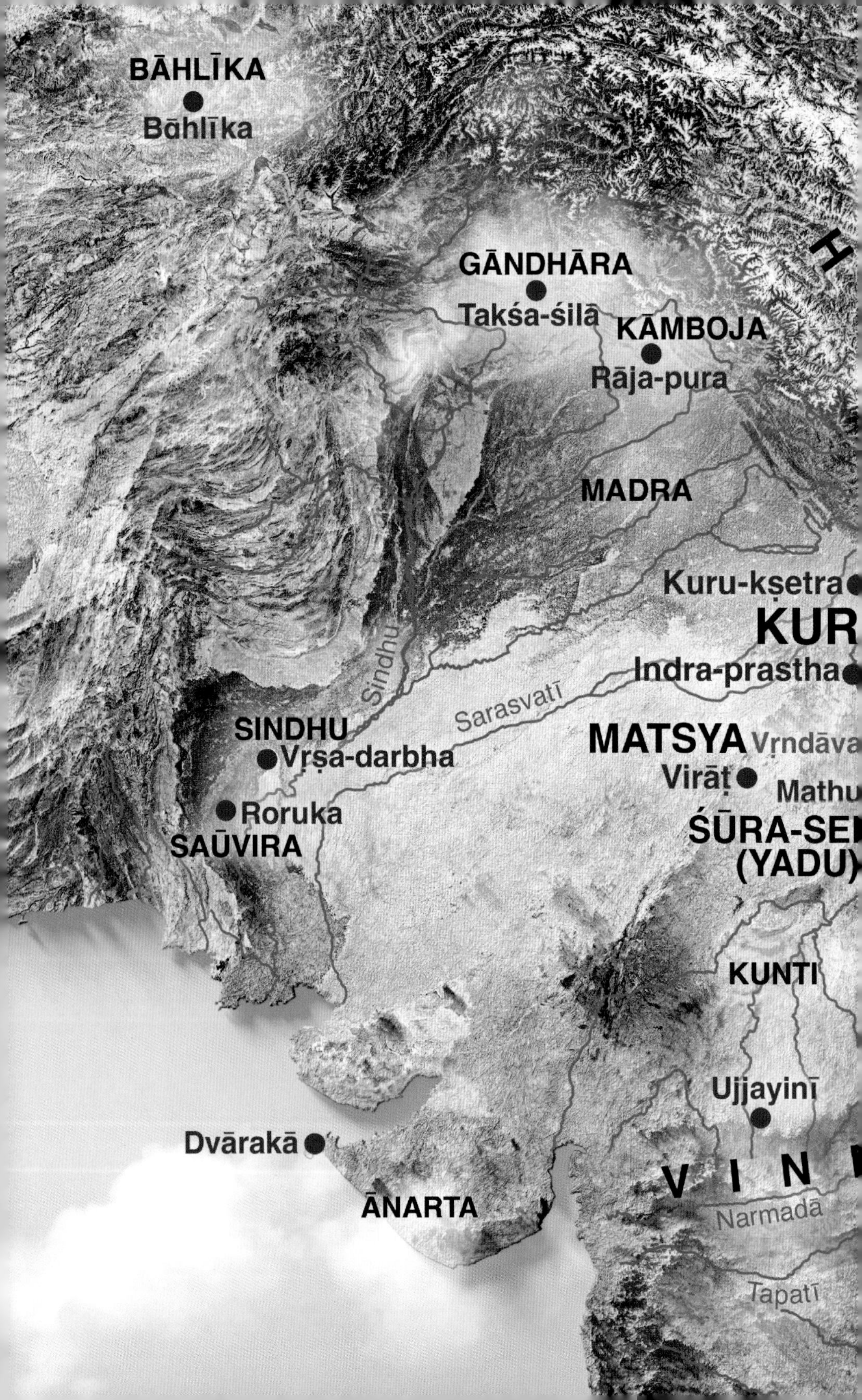
BĀHLĪKA
Bāhlīka
H
GĀNDHĀRA
Takśa-śilā
KĀMBOJA
Rāja-pura
MADRA
Kuru-kṣetra
KUR
Indra-prastha
Sindhu
Sarasvatī
SINDHU
Vṛṣa-darbha
MATSYA
Vṛndāva
Virāṭ
Mathu
Roruka
SAŪVIRA
ŚŪRA-SE
(YADU)
KUNTI
Ujjayinī
Dvārakā
V I N
ĀNARTA
Narmadā
Tapatī

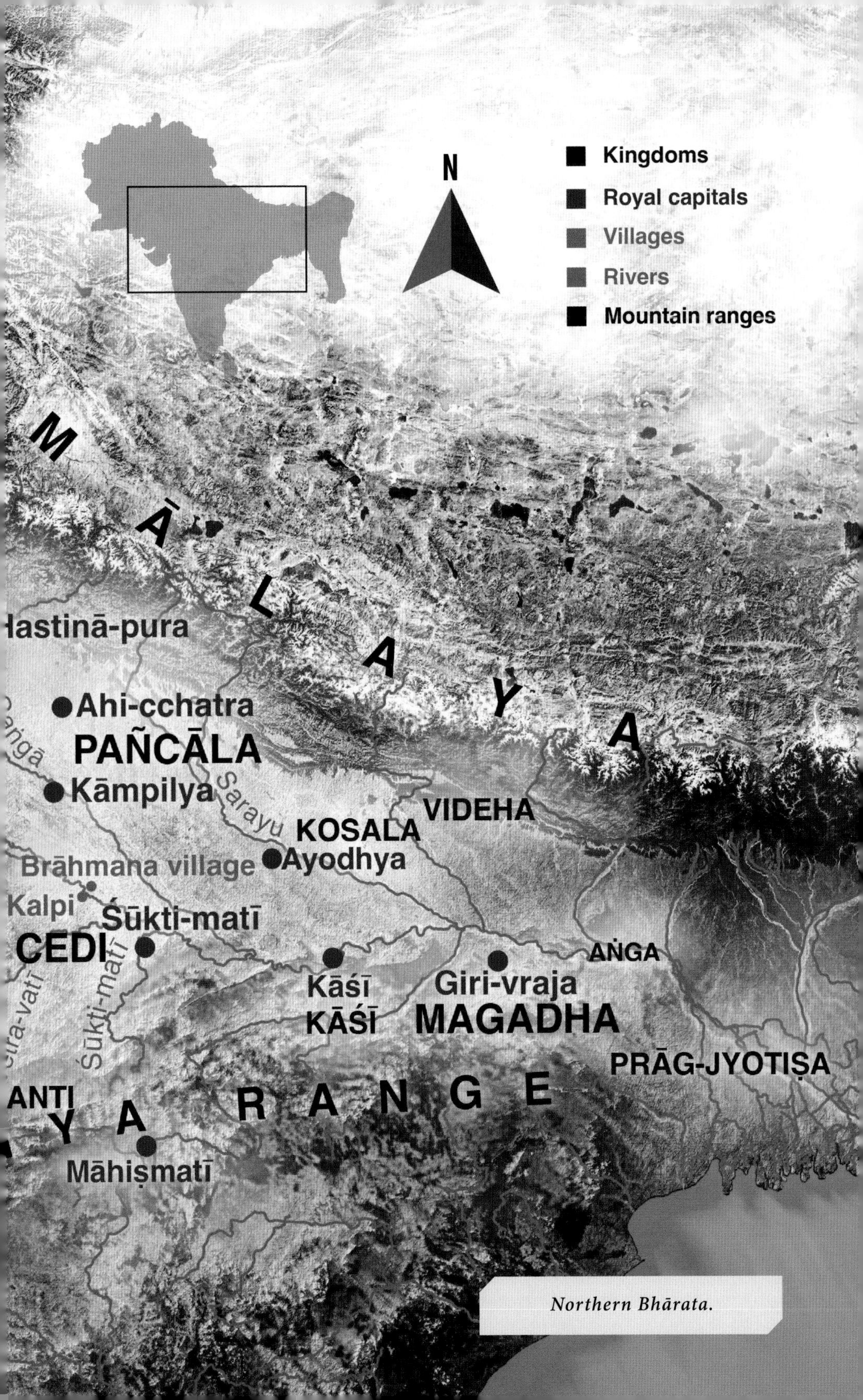

Northern Bhārata.

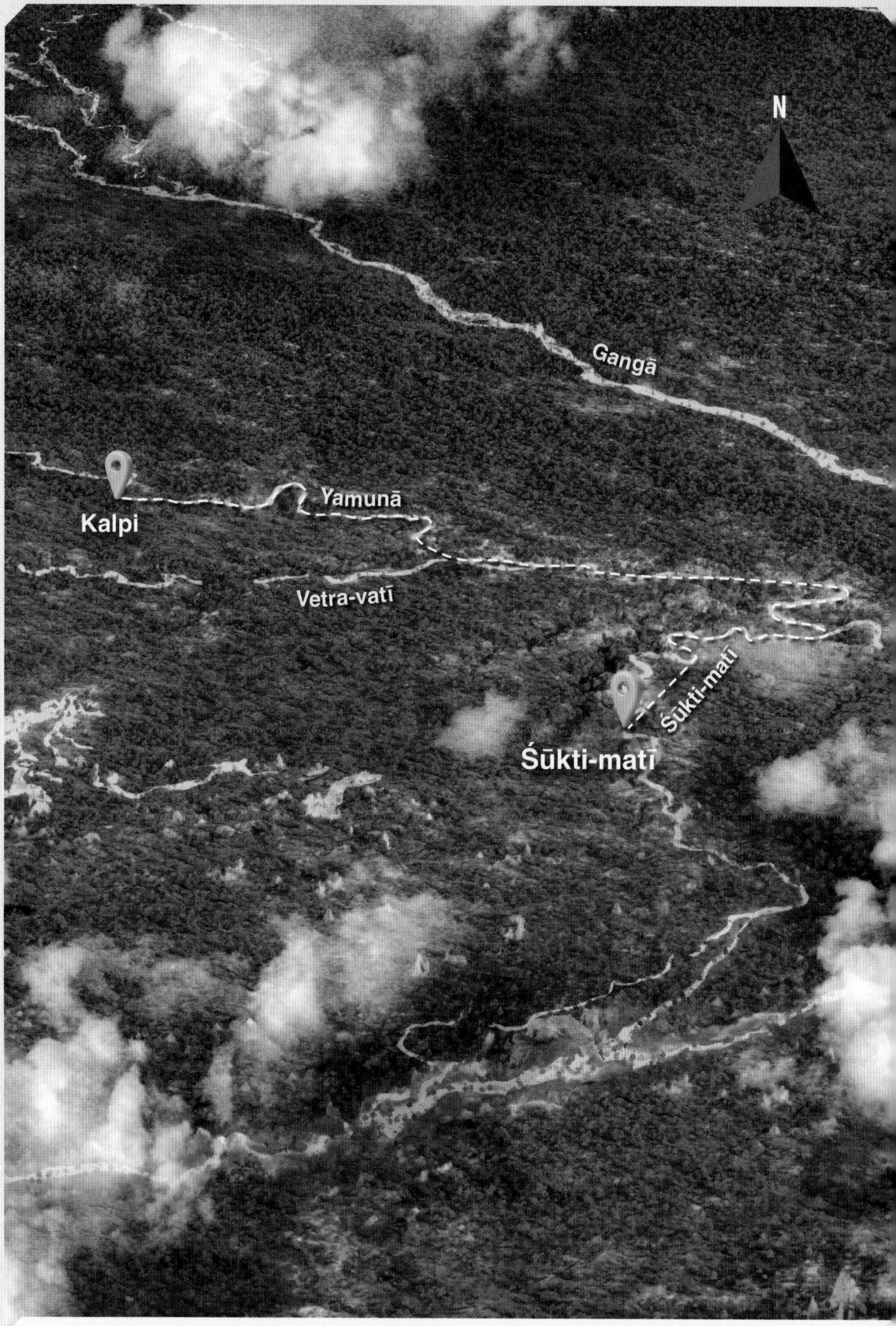

Satya-vatī's journey from Kalpi to Śukti-matī (Pearl River).

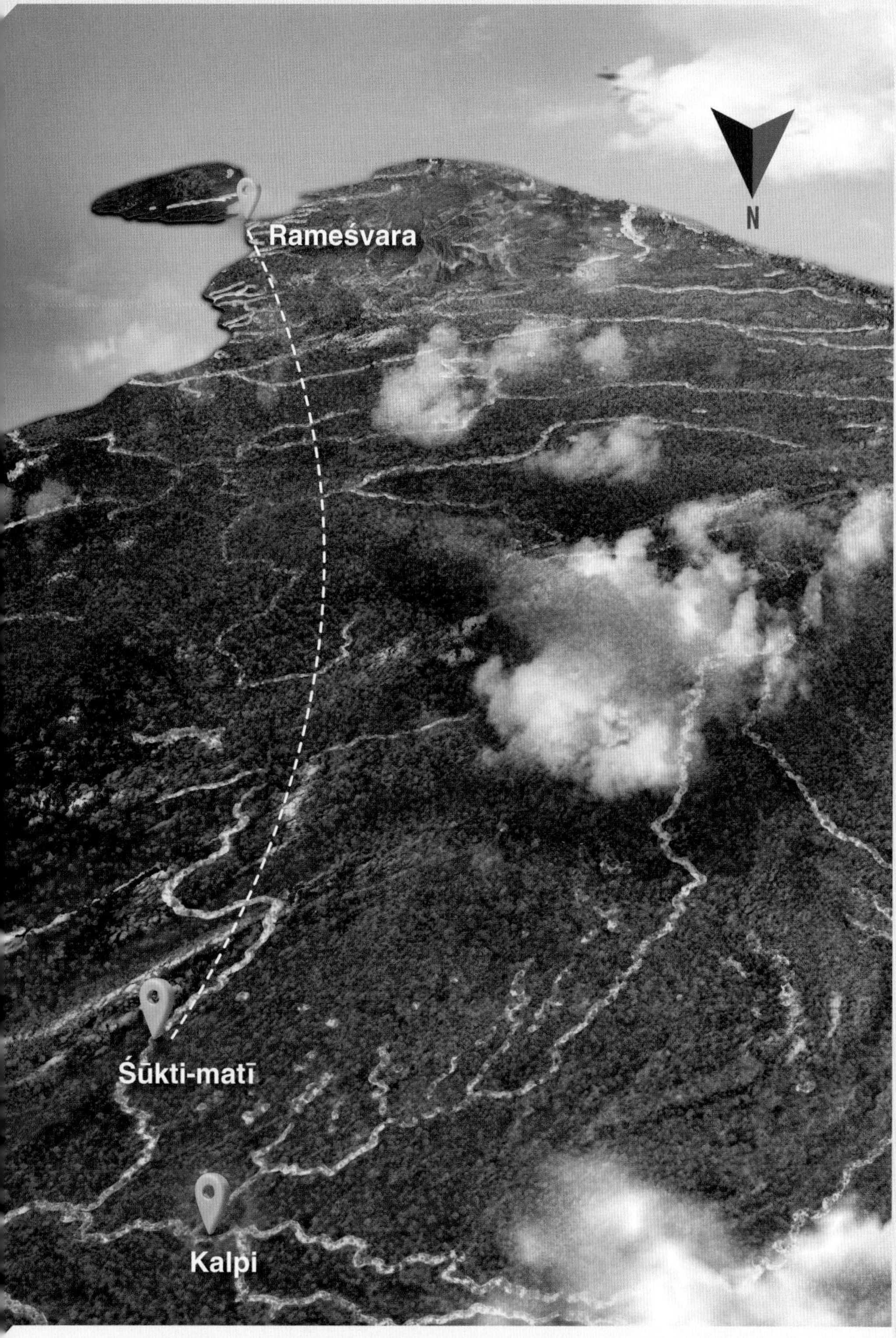

Satya-vatī and her royal family fly from Śukti-matī to Rameśvara.

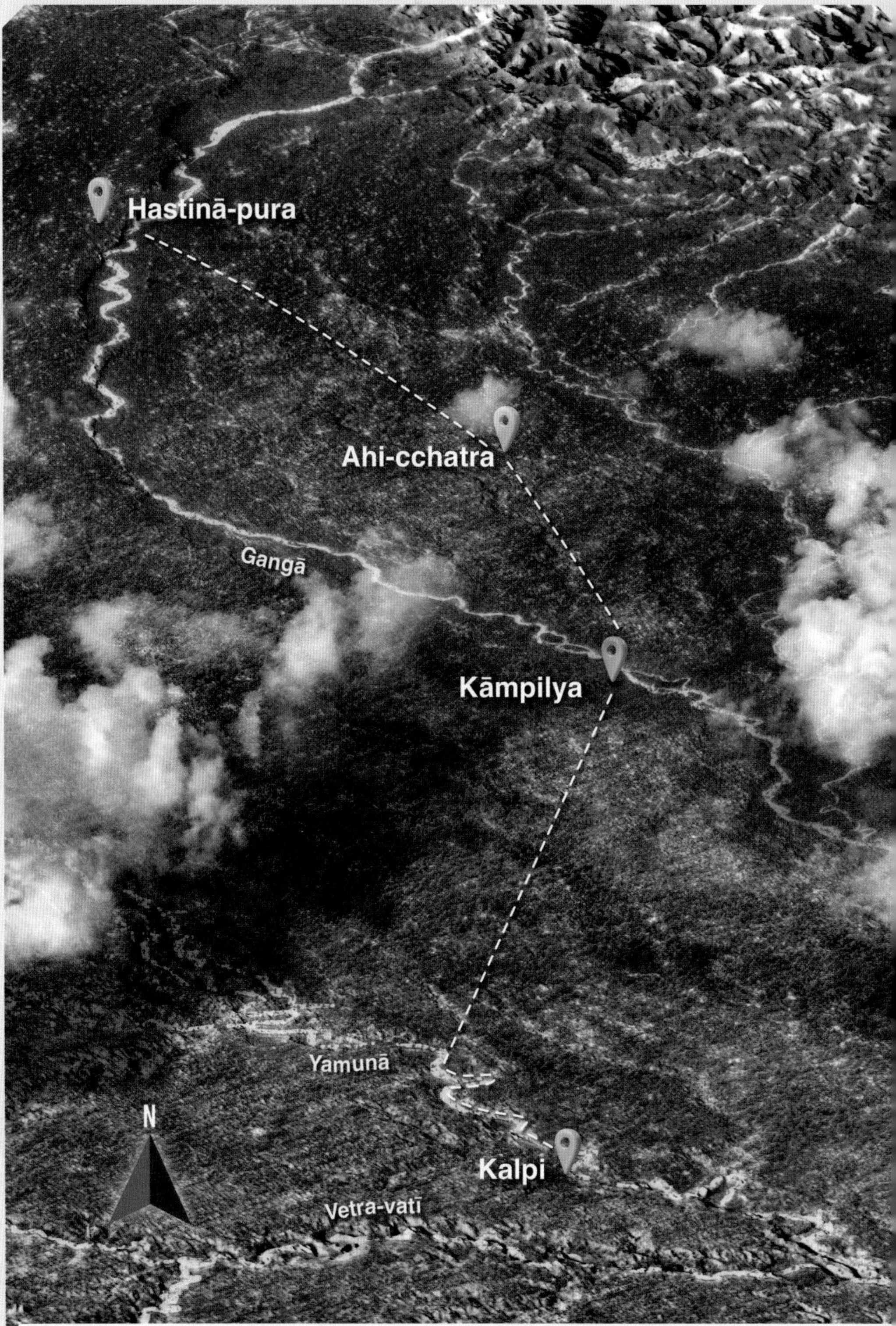

Satya-vatī's journey from Kalpi to Śukti-matī (Pearl River).

CHAPTER 5

Honoring sage Nārada's words, Indra and the Devas lowered their weapons. They begged leave of Nārada and departed for the worlds they each rule.

Back on the Milk Shore, where lapping waves turn sand to emeralds, the Asuras found themselves strangely alone. Anxious to leave lest Devas return, battered Asura survivors, carrying fallen comrades, staggered and stumbled toward Sunset Mountain at the order of their powerful guru Śukra. Vipra-citti personally carried Kāla-nemi's lifeless body.

As they approached the high mountain, darkened by shadows, the Asuras looked up and gazed in wonder at the dark green peak that rose high above the scattered clouds. Crystalline creeks rushed and glided down the slopes, interlacing and moving apart, only to intertwine again farther down the slope.

Ascending the mountain, carrying their revivable dead, the Asuras reached a broad plateau just below the peak. There, in an alpine meadow, circled by clear, moving waters, stood mighty Śukra, the guru of the Asuras. As the dead were laid in rows before him, he walked up and down the rows, looking, nodding, rubbing his hands. He began to apply his saṃ-jīvanī power, which could bring a living soul back to a dead body whose head, neck, and limbs were intact.

Kāla-nemi, the first to be revived, sat up, shook his head, and slowly climbed to his feet. Flexing his huge arms, recalling his violent death at Viṣṇu's hand, the mighty Asura shook with rage. Vipra-citti embraced him. The two friends bowed to Śukra, who was busily engaged reviving other Asuras.

When all the eligible Asuras regained their life, and sat before their guru, he said sternly, "I hope you see the mistake that led to your defeat. You invoked Dark

Magic, and that provoked Viṣṇu. Had you followed me strictly, and paid heed to Dharma, Viṣṇu would not have come, and you might have won. We must prepare with greater discipline for the next battle."

Standing in the back, huge forearms crossed and resting on his immense chest, Kāla-nemi said, "My teacher, I am eternally in debt to you for bringing me back into this body. Whatever I conquer in the three worlds shall be yours to enjoy. But I cannot follow your plan."

The Asura guru clenched his fists. "Do you dare defy me?"

The other Asuras looked on with astonishment at Kāla-nemi. No Asura had ever defied powerful Śukra.

"Control your protégé," Śukra warned Vipra-citti, "before my anger undoes him." Śukra lifted his staff menacingly.

Vipra-citti bowed his head. "Forgive him, dear Śukra, he means you no offense. But with much respect, I say that we can no longer follow the same policy. I beg you, do not hate or harm us. But we are determined to rule the three worlds, and we will never do so as long as Viṣṇu lives."

"Exactly," Kāla-nemi growled. "Our real problem is Viṣṇu."

"Yes," said Śukra haughtily, "and Viṣṇu will continue to be your problem, but I shall not help you." Śukra turned his back to the Asuras and began to walk away.

Kāla-nemi ran after him, calling out, "O Master. I am forever grateful to you for bringing me back to life in this same body. I hold you in highest regard. But I will kill Viṣṇu. And as Vipra-citti said, we know how to rob him of his power and end him forever."

Vipra-citti rushed up to Śukra and said, "Master, he is right, I assure you. We know how to kill Viṣṇu."

"And how will you do that?" Śukra asked with contempt, keeping his back to the Asuras.

Vipra-citti spoke confidently, making dramatic gestures with his massive hands. "Surely you've seen, master, that Earth is Viṣṇu's special little planet. He protects it in every age. He gives special attention to the brāhmaṇas there, many of whom are devoted to him. But why would Viṣṇu give so much attention and care to that little planet? Why would he do that?"

"What are you talking about?" Śukra demanded.

"I mean this," Vipra-citti replied, nodding confidently. "One always hears that Viṣṇu protects the sages, that he empowers them. But the truth is just the opposite. In fact, as you always taught us, Guru Śukra, power lies in mastering the sheer mechanism of the cosmos. That mastery manifests in the process of yajña, the great offering, which bends cosmic forces into cycles of reciprocation with one who masters the process. The master of yajña draws from the universe great power that can be channeled at one's will. Viṣṇu's brāhmaṇas channel cosmic force into Viṣṇu. That, and that alone, is the source of his power. That is precisely why Viṣṇu gives such inordinate attention to little Earth, defending it and protecting its brāhmaṇas. Isn't it clear? A group of advanced brāhmaṇas stays on that small planet, Earth, producing immense power for Viṣṇu. They are fanatically loyal to him. They even call themselves Vaiṣṇavas, devotees of Viṣṇu."

"Very clever," Śukra said with a contemptuous laugh, keeping his back to the Asuras. "So, what is your plan?"

"Here is the plan," Vipra-citti said. "We will eliminate Viṣṇu's brāhmaṇas and thus cut off his power forever."

"What do you mean, eliminate Viṣṇu's brāhmaṇas?" Śukra asked.

"I mean we shall invade Earth and kill those brāhmaṇas. Viṣṇu loses his source of power. He weakens. And then we kill Viṣṇu."

Śukra spun around with burning eyes, facing the Asuras. "You are all mad!" he cried. "You dare to speak of killing brāhmaṇas? My father, mighty Bhṛgu, the first brāhmaṇa, warned me not to help you. He told me you were wicked. But I thought I knew better. I thought the Devas had unfairly rejected you, that you were victims of their discrimination, and that I could help you. But I was wrong. Do you think I would ever help you to kill brāhmaṇas, when I myself am a brāhmaṇa?"

Vipra-citti boldly looked into Śukra's eyes. "In fact, we never believed you would help us in this plan."

With icy repugnance, Śukra said calmly, "You know that the Law ruins those who offend it. Surely you know the price you will pay for these heinous acts."

"Oh, we will not commit heinous acts," Vipra-citti said. "Some of us will take birth on Earth as savage animals. Many of Viṣṇu's brāhmaṇas renounce the world and live in the forest. They will be easy prey. You have always taught us that a wild beast does not offend Dharma when it behaves like a wild beast. Those were your words."

In the past, whenever Śukra threatened to leave them, the Asuras would beg him to stay, promising to do all he asked. But this time, Vipra-citti boldly answered his guru, saying, "With all respect, dear Guru, some of us will no longer submit to a philosophy that we do not really believe. Śukra, we know how the universe functions. It is simply a mechanism inhabited by conscious beings who go from body to body, life after life. There is no absolute truth, no supreme ruler. We have the ability to learn universal laws, master them, and rule the cosmos. Dharma itself is merely a cosmic force. We will study it, master it, and use it for our purpose. We will not blindly obey any law, not even Dharma. And so, with immense gratitude to you, Śukra, with all respect, I and those who stand with me now set out on our own path."

Śukra shook his head with disgust. "After all I did. I brought you back from death. No more! I will never revive you again." Śukra continued to speak with cool-burning rage. Then he turned and departed, followed by a number of Asuras who were afraid to fight without him. With dark, threatening looks, and knowing nods of future rewards, Vipra-citti held most of the Asuras on his side, though many feared their fate without Śukra.

When Śukra had gone, Vipra-citti stood tall on high ground, and with his fearless voice and mien assured the doubtful of victory.

"There are many brāhmaṇas on Earth," he said, "whom we can easily entice with generous gifts and praise. They will expertly ply the yajña-fire for us. Dear Asuras, thank you for your trust in me! We shall rule the three worlds. Have no doubt."

Asuras erupted in bold, confident shouts. Vipra-citti thanked them, glanced at Kāla-nemi, and said, "Asura brothers, even as I speak, Viṣṇu lounges on his White Island, mocking and despising us, laughing at our dead."

Kāla-nemi shook Sunset Mountain with his roar. "I shall kill Viṣṇu!" he raged. "I shall have my revenge! Tell me what I must do."

"Exactly what I wished to hear," Vipra-citti said, clapping his protégé's shoulder. "Hear now my plan." He looked at each Asura face and said, "Earth lives in a time of peace and plenty. Its kings sit and meditate like yogīs. They are naive, unsuspecting. We shall easily conquer them. And with that planet as our base, we shall conquer the three worlds."

An Asura shouted, "Earth's proud warriors will fight us, and we will have human bodies. Do you see danger there?"

"You don't understand." Vipra-citti smiled. "We will not usurp Earth's kingdoms. We shall inherit them."

Asuras clamored for clarification, some jumping to their feet, others twisting in their seats. Vipra-citti stroked his silken locks with mighty hands, smiled at Kāla-nemi, and said, "Everyone assumes that a mighty Asura would never deign to assume an Earthly body, and indeed, in normal times it would be for us a degradation. But to serve our cause, we will do what we must. We shall deign to take birth on Earth, in the mightiest royal families. In time, and importantly, in full accord with Dharma, we shall inherit the leading kingdoms of Earth and rule that planet, all by the Law."

Here Vipra-citti laughed. "Can you not see the precious irony of it all? The Avatāra Viṣṇu has sworn to protect Dharma. He will thus be forced to protect our right to inherit the Earth. And as we slay his personal brāhmaṇas, those who empower him, he will grow weak as we grow stronger. Seeing this, Viṣṇu will attack us, but in a weakened state, and we shall slay him."

"Brilliant," said a thoughtful Asura. "But once we begin to assert our power, other kings will oppose us. We will fight them in our human bodies. Human bodies are weak."

"Yes. But even in human bodies, we shall retain much Asura power. We will be far stronger than ordinary humans. Earth's kings love to battle each other, to show their strength. And to fight when attacked is a warrior's Dharma. So, following Dharma, we shall destroy rival kings, take their realms, and inherit the rest. Before long, the planet shall be ours. We will then use Earth as a base to conquer the three worlds. Lovely plans."

"But I still fear Dharma's wrath on us if we kill brāhmaṇas," an Asura said.

"Yes." Vipra-citti smiled. "We all know Dharma's power. But remember what I said. When feral beast kills forest sage, it breaks no Law. After all, to kill is surely the Dharma of beasts."

"So you mean…" one Asura began.

"Precisely," said Vipra-citti. "On that remote, little planet where Viṣṇu's brāhmaṇas thrive, chosen Asuras will take birth as deadly beasts and kill forest sages who have the bad habit of using cosmic fire to empower Viṣṇu."

Vipra-citti raised a powerful hand and turned it around to silence any further questions. The jeweled rings on his fingers glowed, reflecting the eerie light of the precious stones that studded Sunset Mountain.

The Asuras fell silent. Vipra-citti nodded in approval. "Listen! We shall descend to Earth in disciplined groups, by generations. I will personally lead our first so-called human generation on Earth. Those Asuras who will take birth as powerful beasts will come at that time. You, Kāla-nemi, will follow us in the next generation. I shall prepare the planet for you." Kāla-nemi nodded, desperate to avenge his defeat.

The Asuras departed Sunset Mountain, winding their way down its mystic slope. They passed a perpetually shaded valley, lit only by self-glowing jewels that adorned its surrounding slopes. In that valley, nine or ten Asura yogīs sat or stood in most difficult postures, unmoving, fully fixed in meditation.

A young Asura called out to the others, "Who are those yogīs? What are they doing here?"

The chilling voice of Kāla-nemi replied. "Those are my trained assassins. They are acquiring immense yoga power. They will help me kill the Avatāra, should he dare come to Earth."

CHAPTER 6

Sitting erect in deep meditation, Satya-vatī gasped. Gone was the celestial battlefield! Sunset Mountain with its plotting Asuras had vanished! She opened her eyes and found herself, as before, sitting in the brāhmaṇa village, facing young sage Parā-śara. He had carried her to the celestial realm and shown her dramatic past events whose outcome would determine the fate of the three worlds.

Sitting on the familiar grassy bank of dear Yamunā, Satya sighed. Parā-śara nodded to her. She could not contain herself. "Oh, Parā-śara! Of all the wonders you showed me, greatest was the vision of Viṣṇu himself! I did not see him clearly. His effulgence was too great. But I knew it was Viṣṇu. I knew it absolutely within my heart."

"Yes. Viṣṇu resides in his abode, but also within our hearts. That's why the greatest yogīs seek him within themselves."

"Thank you. But, Parā-śara! What my father said was true! The Asuras have been killing Viṣṇu's devoted sages. But King Vasu...what has he done?"

"King Vasu has been tirelessly flying all over the world in his crystal aircraft, killing these strange beasts. He saved countless sages. But some died, and died horribly. It breaks our heart. But even that great king, and his brave sons, can't be everywhere at once. I must be honest and tell you that the number of brāhmaṇas devoted to Viṣṇu has decreased. Some have died, and others are afraid to serve Viṣṇu."

Satya-vatī gasped. "But will Viṣṇu still come?"

"Only Viṣṇu knows that."

"Oh Parā-śara! What if the Asuras are right and the universe is simply a sophisticated mechanism that can be understood and controlled? What if the

Asuras succeed? It seems impossible, but what if they defeat Viṣṇu, and seize the three worlds? How will any of us live under their tyranny? I will drown myself at once in dear Yamunā before I submit to the Asuras."

Parā-śara shook his head slowly. "Satya, the Veda says that Viṣṇu is beyond the power of this world."

"Yes, but the Asuras do not accept the Veda. I don't want to doubt Viṣṇu. I know he is very great. But I worry. Here in this village, the brāhmaṇas devote their offerings to Viṣṇu. If Asura beasts attack here, I'm sure our king will protect them. Forgive me for troubling you with my questions, but I must ask you something."

The sage nodded. "Of course."

Satya-vatī looked at him earnestly. "Did King Vasu really get his power, and his famous crystal aircraft, from Indra himself? No other king on Earth could have saved so many sages."

Parā-śara smiled. "I was just about to explain those very topics. Listen carefully and you will again see all that I say."

Satya-vatī folded her hands and bowed to the sage. Parā-śara smiled and began to speak. Satya saw it all, as if she were there.

"Mighty King Vasu was not always powerful and happy. Indeed, as a young prince, he was rather sad and disappointed. He was born in the mighty Kuru dynasty, but into a secondary branch. There were more princes than kingdoms to rule. So, young Vasu inherited only the emblems and insignias of royalty, not the power to do great good, as he fervently wished. For he had no kingdom, no way to engage his exceptional abilities, no chance to fulfill his dreams. Moreover, the world was peaceful and prosperous, so there was little for this heroic prince to do."

"I can see him through your words," Satya-vatī said. "He is quite a handsome young prince, but he does indeed look lonely and sad."

"Yes, and Prince Vasu was also lonely because he did not find a princess he could love. He would not marry without love. Perhaps in that sense, the prince was much like you."

"What do you mean?" Satya asked with a deep blush, riveted to Parā-śara's words.

"I mean only this," he replied. "When we cannot truly be ourselves in the world, nor be with someone we love with heart and mind, we may be lonely even when surrounded by many people."

Satya-vatī again blushed. How did the sage know her so well? And how could she, a fisherman's daughter, resemble a Kuru prince?

"What did Prince Vasu do?" Satya asked anxiously.

"He gave up all hope of finding love or purpose in this world. So, several years before your birth, Prince Vasu put down his weapons, renounced his opulent life, and retired to the deep forest, to an āśrama as lonely as his heart."

Satya-vatī gasped. "I see it all," she said, eyes closed in meditation. "The prince went deep into the wilderness."

"Yes. There he fixed his mind on a higher world he might achieve through mystic yoga practice. He aimed for Indra-loka, the fabulous world of Indra, lord of the Devas. Of course you saw that celestial sphere."

Satya-vatī nodded.

"And so," Parā-śara continued, "this determined prince poured his fierce warrior resolve into his yoga practice. He delighted in austerity, and conquered not other warriors but his own senses and desires. On rare occasions when other yogīs visited that secluded hermitage, the prince's power and determination astounded them."

"I too admire that prince," Satya-vatī said. "I admire him greatly. He preserved his autonomy and dignity. He found a situation where he could at least rule himself, and not be subject to the whims of others. Indeed, he was not even subject to the whims of his own body. He the soul ruled the body."

"So," Parā-śara said, "you know about the soul."

"Oh yes," Satya said. "I've spent so many years serving the sages and listening to their talks. They taught me all about the true self."

"Of course," the sage said. "They are wise and kind. They do credit to the brāhmaṇa order. But I shall continue my story."

"Yes, please do."

Parā-śara nodded. "So assiduously did the prince follow his path that he would soon reach Indra's celestial realm. But then something unprecedented happened. Indra himself, lord of the Devas, came to Earth to see the prince!"

"Indra himself? Here on Earth?"

"Yes. As I said, it was unprecedented. The prince could hardly believe his eyes. As described in the Veda, and as you have seen, Indra's hair and complexion shone with the golden hue of sunshine. He held his Vajra weapon that shoots indomitable lightning, as it did in the battle against the Asuras."

"Yes," Satya whispered, eager to hear more. Eyes closed, carried on Parā-śara's words, she saw Prince Vasu bow and say to the Deva leader, "Lord Indra, you honor me greatly by your visit to my poor hermitage. How may I serve you?"

Indra replied. "O prince, I know of your disappointment and pain, and why you came to this wilderness. You have indeed earned your passage to my world."

Joyful, the prince assumed that Indra had come to escort him to that celestial world, though he did not grasp why the great Deva would personally come for that. But the prince quickly learned that Indra came with a very different purpose.

Pacing in front of the prince, deep in thought, Indra turned to face him and said, "Despite your merit, Vasu, or more accurately because of it, I ask you to remain on Earth and finish your natural life here."

Vasu's heart sank at these words. He pleaded, "Lord Indra, in my heart, I already gave up the Earth. There is nothing for me here."

"Oh but there is," Indra said with a knowing smile. The noon sun shone brightly on the Deva's golden hair. He looked on the downcast prince with amused sympathy. "In the future, Vasu, you will achieve higher worlds. But for now, protect the Earth, as I protect the worlds above."

Vasu looked up at the Deva and said, "Protect the Earth? From what, Lord Indra? I ask with great respect. You know that Earth flourishes. The citizens are happy and safe. We truly live a golden age since Paraśu-rāma slew the wicked kings. As you know, saintly kings born of brāhmaṇa fathers rule everywhere. Even the Kuru monarch Pratīpa sits like a grand yogī on the bank of sacred Gaṅgā and meditates on the world's welfare. O Indra, this world needs no defender. Even you, my lord, show your pleasure with Earth by sending rain at the best times and places, sustaining all creatures. It is truly a golden age. Please, let me go to your world."

"I understand your feelings," Indra said. "I shall now explain mine. With Viṣṇu's aid, we Devas won our battle with the Asuras. We did not win the war. The Asura guru Śukra brought the slain Asuras back to life. They will attack again."

"Won't Viṣṇu stop them again?"

"Perhaps. This time the Asuras will attack with greater cunning."

Indra then explained the Asura strategy, as articulated in Sunset Mountain, including the attacks on Viṣṇu's brāhmaṇas.

Vasu's shock was visible in every feature of his face. "Yet no one on Earth suspects that Asuras walk among us. We see only peace and prosperity."

Indra smiled and shook his head. "How little you people of Earth understand your danger. You are like babes sleeping in a garden as a tiger stalks you. Asuras are slowly invading your planet, undetected by any of you. The Asuras chose your planet precisely because it is so prospering, naive, and unsuspecting. They will soon take birth as princes of royal houses. Thus, without firing a weapon, they will inherit great kingdoms."

Vasu said, "And they really have that power, to take birth where they like?"

"Of course," Indra said. "Remember, the Asuras are half-brothers of the Devas. Their powers are similar to ours."

Astonished, Vasu shivered as cool breezes blew over him. "They will actually attack sages. That is an evil beyond imagination. Even in the bodies of beasts, they know exactly what they are doing. How then can they avoid their guilt?"

"They believe they can. They believe the universe is ultimately a mere mechanism. And they have powers like the Devas."

Vasu's face and body tightened in steely determination. "I will do all I can to help you stop the Asuras. I will gladly abandon my ascetic practice and celestial ambition and fight for this noble cause. But how can I help? I am alone in the world."

Indra smiled. "I will give special power to a royal dynasty that will defend Dharma on this planet. I have chosen you to lead that dynasty. Of course, you must accept."

Stunned by this offer, Prince Vasu stood motionless. Indra smiled again and said, "If you do protect Dharma from the Asuras, Dharma will protect you. And in your next life, you will have your choice of worlds in which to reside."

"Is this really happening?" said the startled prince.

"Yes, it is. I offer you my friendship. Protect the world on my behalf. Become my friend, and I shall be a friend to you."

Prince Vasu, still astonished, stammered, "Of course, Lord Indra, I wish to be your friend. That is a great honor for me. But how will I fight mighty Asuras? At present I have no kingdom, no army."

Indra laughed. "Oh, I will fix that. I shall make you the emperor of the world."

Prince Vasu's eyebrows shot up and he gasped. "An emperor? Lord Indra, for generations, imperial power has rested with the Kurus of Hastinā-pura. Noble Pratīpa rules there. I am not his heir."

"Yes, the Kurus of Hastinā-pura have long protected this world. But peace and plenty have created a false confidence among kings. The Kuru lord, Pratīpa, sits and meditates, praying for the good of all creatures. He is righteous, to be sure, but unprepared to fight an Asura invasion. Dire circumstances call for special measures. You shall be king of kings, but you will need an imperial seat. Therefore, I shall grant you the excellent kingdom of Cedi."

Vasu's eyes opened wide. "Cedi? It is indeed a rich and mighty realm. But Cedi has a ruler. I cannot usurp his throne. I would offend Dharma, as you well know. Granting that your words must come true, and I somehow become Cedi's king, no ruler on Earth will recognize me as king of kings."

Great Indra laughed. "Trust me, young prince. You shall be king of Cedi, and emperor of the world. And we will not offend Dharma in the process."

The astonished young prince again bowed and assured Indra of his trust. The Deva lord said, "Cedi is an excellent country. It abounds in lovely lakes, hills, rivers, and forests – all that Earth offers. Its people are virtuous. They do not lie, even in jest. Cedi boasts a formidable army that you will lead. Indeed, my friend, Cedi surpasses other realms in its virtue, beauty, and treasure."

"But what will I do, my lord, when I become Cedi's ruler? Shall I march with the Cedi army against the Asura princes?"

Indra shook his head. "No, not now. For now, you can defend the brāhmaṇas. I will give you special power for that. We cannot oppose Asura princes yet, for they are still consolidating their power and have broken no Law. We too must follow Dharma or we will lose our own power."

Still wracked by doubts, Prince Vasu wanted to ask, "How will I fight Asuras with superhuman powers?" But fearing he would try Indra's patience, he kept his head bowed and said nothing.

Indra seemed to read his mind. "I will grant you extraordinary martial power. When they see your power, all the world's monarchs, those that are not Asuras, shall honor and follow you."

Vasu wondered what form that martial power would take. Again, Indra replied to his thoughts. "I will grant you a military aircraft like those of the Devas. It is a large crystal aircraft, with palatial comforts. This silent craft moves at unfathomable speed, and will be guided by your will alone. It will fly to any place on Earth, and with it, you will fight the Asuras. I will grant you other powers as well, but use them only to protect the innocent. And we must not panic the world. Speak of the Asura invasion only to your wife, and later to your sons."

"My wife? Sons?"

"Yes, you will learn about that soon enough. You may also speak the truth to those who are devoted to Viṣṇu. Just remember, your world is in grave danger. I have chosen you to protect it. Always act as my friend, obey my instructions, and you will be victorious."

"I shall obey," the prince said with a bow. "I am most grateful."

Indra nodded. In a grave tone, he gave the prince final instructions. "You renounced the pleasures of this world. In that same spirit of detachment, you must serve the world as a great king. You must never use imperial power to exploit others. Serve the world unselfishly. Your success, your glory, depends on it. Rule as a form of spiritual yoga, without pride or vanity, and you will succeed."

Prince Vasu bowed, and assured Indra that his instructions would be faithfully followed.

Indra nodded. "Go now to Cedi. Do not doubt my words."

"I have no doubt," Vasu said, saluting the Deva lord.

As Prince Vasu gazed in wonder, and marveled at all that Indra had said, the Deva lord rose into the sky. Looking down at Vasu, he said in a voice as deep as thunder, "So be it, prince. Go to Cedi now." At once, Indra vanished. Vasu remained there for some time staring at that place in the sky where he last saw Indra. What would the prince do now. He knew not the way to Cedi. Even if he found his way there, why would a proud nation accept as their king, a man who looked like an emaciated beggar?

CHAPTER 7

On the bank of the Yamunā River, in a village of brāhmaṇas, Satya-vatī opened her eyes in wonder. She looked at Parā-śara, who had paused his narration. He smiled at her, and suggested that she stand up and stretch, after sitting so long in meditation.

Exhilarated, astonished, she rose to her feet, stretched her arms and back, and walked about the forest to calm herself. After several minutes, she returned to Parā-śara and said, "O sage, I am eager to hear. Please tell me more, unless of course you wish to rest."

"I am happy to continue," he said. "Let us follow Prince Vasu to Cedi."

"Oh yes!" cried Satya-vatī, resuming her yoga āsana, and expectantly waiting for Parā-śara's words. He began.

Prince Vasu could not imagine how he was to become king of Cedi. Why would the citizens of Cedi accept him? But then Indra's thundering words echoed in the sky. Go to Cedi now!

Sighing deeply, running his fingers through his wavy hair, the handsome prince cast aside his incredulity and swung into action. Chanting mantras, he extinguished the sacred fire into which he had made daily offerings. He had never intended to return to civilization on this planet, and had no belongings but the ragged cloth that covered him. "I will travel light," he joked to himself.

Guided only by sun, moon, and stars, he must labor his way through wild and dense forest, in the general direction of Cedi. It would be a long journey. Eventually, he must come to some village or other. There he would ask directions.

But no sooner had Prince Vasu taken his first steps than a forest path, covered in soft, cropped grass, opened before him, a path that was not there before. Indra was truly guiding him.

The prince had spent the last few years in austerity, giving his emaciated body just enough food and water to support his meditation. But new energy filled him. Indeed, as he walked, power filled his limbs. Clarity filled his mind.

Eager to test his new powers, he grabbed a stone and hurled it an impossible distance with startling precision. Great Indra had indeed empowered him. Vasu could not doubt the rest.

After days of travel, wilderness transformed into lush farms, with neat rows of peas, cauliflower, okra, eggplant, beans, and many other vegetables. Varieties of rice, wheat, multicolored millets, and other grains grew in lush abundance.

Black pepper, cinnamon, turmeric, cardamom, sugar cane, mustard, sesame, betel-nut, ginger, and cumin all painted the landscape in bright, geometric colors that flashed in the bright sun.

Wide fields of flowers in radiant colors carpeted swaths of countryside. The heady fragrance of rose, jasmine, champa, and other flowers thrilled the weary traveler.

A sparkling, liquid lattice of rivers, streams, and channels fed crystalline currents to thirsty, many-hued orchards, laden with bananas, mangoes, jackfruit, berries, and myriad other fruits. Even common farm workers dressed well in fine, airy cotton, with plentiful ornaments of gold and semi-precious stones.

Reaching a particularly prosperous village, he confirmed that he had entered the kingdom of Cedi. As Indra had told, the people were kind, affluent, virtuous. These free citizens lived under constitutional monarchy in which every citizen, whether beggar or monarch, must obey Dharma, sacred Law. These free people might soon be ruled by Asura tyrants, yet Indra's command, and Vasu's own good sense, forbade him from revealing the perilous state of their land.

Absorbed in observation and deep reflection, he reached the outskirts of Cedi's splendid capital, Pearl River, in less time than he thought possible. He gazed upon the handsome homes, surrounded by leafy gardens that lined well-shaded avenues. Spacious plazas, paved in fine tiles and cooled by shooting fountains, embellished the crossings. In the city center stood a lofty marble palace of exquisite design, tastefully trimmed in gold. This was Pearl River, the great Cedi capital.

He admired the fine dress of the citizens, and their healthy bodies adorned with jewels and gold. Still dressed in a yogī's rags, he was unnerved by the frequent stares. He was greatly out of place. Yet he was to be king of this land. Oh Indra, he thought, what is to happen now?

How could he possibly assume the Cedi throne? The people were all kind, but no one seemed to take him seriously, other than finding the sudden appearance of a ragged yogi in the middle of the city to be most unusual. He had renounced his wealth and owned nothing, not even a sword or a bow. He had only Indra's word that he, Vasu, was to rule this mighty, opulent realm of Cedi.

What was he to do? Perhaps he should knock on the palace door and explain that he was Cedi's new king. He laughed at the idea. For now, he stayed in the city center where the royal palace loomed above lovely Pearl River.

Suddenly, with a heart-stopping thunderclap, heavy rain rushed down. As he sought shelter, the downpour drenched him. Mud splattered him. He sighed. He had never looked worse, never so wretched and dirty. Indra, god of thunder and rain, had sent him a personal welcome.

Still, the sun darted and flashed through the tropical rain clouds. Spying shelter, Prince Vasu dashed under an artfully carved arcade, built of red sandstone that glistened in the rain and sun. Waiting for the rain to cease, he noticed a large hill rising behind the river. A friendly merchant, sheltering there, asked, "Young man, are you from the capital?"

"No, sir, this is my first time here," Vasu said.

"Sorry about this unseasonal rain," the man said. "Both its timing, and the sheer quantity of rain, are most unusual for this region."

What luck! Was it actually Indra, or some mischievous spirit of nature?

Looking at the prince's ragged, muddy clothes, the merchant said, "Whoever you may be, welcome to our city. That hill you stare at, behind the river, is Kolā-hala, the uproarious one. You can hear the wind roar by the hill. Some citizens even believe that a dangerous spirit lives within its slopes."

Perhaps those people were right, for the great hill began to groan and shake most strangely. Crowds suddenly ran about the city center, shouting in utter panic and desperation. Vasu strained to decipher their cries.

"Oh Lord!" cried the merchant. "A girl is trapped up on the hill and it's about to split in the storm. It's a landslide! She'll die in the mud or the river. Who can save her?"

The young girl apparently had not feared the malevolent spirit said to inhabit the hill. She had been sitting on a grassy plateau of Mount Kolā-hala, high above the river. Her life was now in grave danger.

Instantly, Prince Vasu raced toward the river. As he ran, he astonished the people and himself by his superhuman speed. But there was no time to think about that now. Reaching the bank, he raced toward that spot directly across the river from the hill. The girl desperately clung to a tree. The riotous hill quaked, roared, and split. A dislodged slab of slope holding the poor girl slid free and plunged into lovely Pearl River, as if to ravish its waters.

Vasu watched in horror as with a cry, the girl fell headlong into the river's deep, seething waters. The waves churned violently as if struggling against the hill's assault.

Vasu would now test his new Indra-given powers. Indeed, he staked his life on them, for he must try to save the girl. He ran to the riverbank and dove into the wild flood.

CHAPTER 8

In a hamlet of sages, on the bank of holy Yamunā, young Satya-vatī cried out in anguish. By the power of Parā-śara's words, she saw a young girl, not much older than herself, thrashing about in the river, as if in her death throes. Parā-śara honored her concern with a bow of his head and continued narrating. Satya-vatī saw it all.

Grasping the still-conscious girl with one arm, and shouting to her through the din to hold onto him — which she somehow did — Vasu fought his way to shore with his other arm, astonished at his own power. Indra had not failed him.

As he emerged from the river, carrying the girl, deafening cheers greeted him from the swelling crowds. Prince Vasu carried the girl to higher ground, placing her gently on soft grass. Her eyes were closed but she breathed.

The rain stopped as quickly as it came, and the tropical sun shone brightly. Vasu gently pushed her silken locks from her lovely face and prayed. She opened her eyes, startled to see a bearded face, with long, tangled hair, staring down at her. She tried to hold him in her gaze, and to thank him, but strength failed her. Vasu entreated her to rest and conserve her energy. She faintly nodded her agreement, parted her lips, and gasped, "Thank you. You saved my life."

He shook his head, told her that God had saved her, and urged her again to conserve her strength. But she would speak. "Who are you?" she whispered faintly.

"I am Prince Vasu, son of Sudhanu, and grandson of great Kuru. And I am your faithful servant. Please rest."

She smiled faintly, and in a barely audible murmur said, "I am honored to meet a Kuru prince. I am Girikā." He smiled and bowed to her. After a minute, an amused smile spread faintly over her face. He looked at her quizzically, and she whispered in a slightly stronger tone, "Prince, forgive me. At this moment, I am unable to offer you a proper royal reception."

Too weak to laugh, her eyes filled with affectionate mirth. The crisis having passed, Vasu observed that she was indeed a very lovely and bright young lady. But before he could say something kind and witty, a platoon of armed royal guards rushed toward them, cleared away onlookers, and signaled physicians, who raced to Girikā.

Vasu obeyed the polite requests that he move back and give room to the medical experts. Quickly ascertaining that her condition was not life-threatening, they administered herbal relaxants, and ordered that she be lifted by guards into a royal chariot.

Becoming drowsy under the power of those herbs, the girl's eyes, before they closed, searched for Vasu. Finding him, she said, "Come to see me," and fell unconscious. Surrounded by female attendants, she was quickly driven toward the city.

A royal minister approached Vasu, who stood gazing at Girikā's swiftly vanishing chariot. With respectful inquiries, which Vasu answered with equal decorum, the minister learned that Vasu was a Kuru prince. With much esteem and gratitude, he thanked Vasu for saving the girl's life. Vasu protested that he had simply done his duty. The minister insisted that Vasu accompany him to the royal palace, and that he stay there as long as he wished as the honored guest of the Queen of Cedi.

Vasu gratefully accepted the invitation, and then said, "Forgive my ignorance, for I have spent several years in the wilderness, engaged in austere yoga. Kindly tell me, who is the queen of Cedi?"

The minister smiled. "You just saved her life. My dear prince, like it or not, you are a national hero in Cedi. News of your most heroic act has surely spread throughout the capital, and by tomorrow, it will be known throughout the nation. For now, I just hope we can get you through the crowds of citizens that are waiting to catch a glimpse of you, and shout their gratitude."

"It was my great honor to serve your noble queen. And the king, her husband?"

"Oh, we have no king, not yet. Many have tried to win her hand, but our Queen Girikā is not easily impressed with young royals."

"I see." Was this Indra's plan? Vasu had barely arrived in Cedi, yet he had already saved the life of its queen, thus becoming a national hero. Further, he suspected, after a very short acquaintance, that he could love the beautiful young queen. But could she love him?

The minister and a military escort somehow brought him through the cheering crowds. He saw that the people of Cedi loved their queen, and they adored the prince who saved her. It must be Indra.

He was taken to the royal palace. Closely encircled by his military escort, and surrounded by large, tumultuous crowds, he hardly saw or noticed anything around him, till he was actually inside the palace.

The minister took him to an opulent suite, finely furnished. His rooms enjoyed extensive natural light and breezes, and opened onto a lush private garden. The minister asked, with no trace of pride or presumption, if these accommodations were adequate. They certainly were. Having spent a few years in a most austere wilderness, Vasu found his quarters in the Cedi palace to be worthy of Indra himself. Finally, the minister opened a closet door and pointed out a wide row of opulent garments that might please the prince. The prince was pleased indeed. His present duty made his ragged yoga garb obsolete.

The minister excused himself, bowed, and left the Kuru prince to bathe and dress. Vasu spent the evening in the balmy, scented air of his personal garden. He wondered how Girikā was recovering, what she was doing, and what she thought of him.

The next morning, handsomely uniformed palace staff brought him a sumptuous breakfast. He went out to walk in the city, but was soon recognized, and had to flee back to the palace as exuberant crowds of admirers quickly gathered. Soon after, a herald came to the door and delivered a message from Queen Girikā. The queen requested the honor of his presence at lunch. He accepted with warm alacrity and eloquent expressions of gratitude.

When he arrived for what looked to be a royal banquet, the young queen gazed at him approvingly. Gone was the disheveled, scruffy, bearded yogī. In his place came an elegant, handsome Kuru prince. Prince Vasu knew that the queen was duly informed of his identity as Kuru royalty.

Girikā was quickly recovering her strength. She greeted Vasu like an old friend, to his great pleasure, and he reciprocated. She offered him earnest and repeated thanks for saving her life. He was honored to have the chance to render service to Her Majesty.

The young royals seemed engaged in a competition of civilities and appreciation. He took his seat facing young Girikā. After light banter at the sumptuous meal, Girikā invited Vasu to her garden, which spread for acres, with manicured, emerald lawns, fruit- and flower-bearing trees, and gently rolling meadows.

Once they were alone, he sincerely inquired about her health. She assured him that the expert prognosis was for a full, rapid recovery.

"I thank Viṣṇu for that," he exclaimed spontaneously.

"By all means," she said, with an inscrutable smile. "Let us thank Viṣṇu."

Did she speak in earnest? Did she accept Viṣṇu as he did, as the highest cosmic authority? Or did she speak mere diplomacy? Worse yet, could lovely Girikā have sympathy for, or be one of, the Asuras? Were her words meant to mislead him, and gain his confidence? He was strongly inclined toward the first thesis, that she truly accepted Viṣṇu. In that case, she might marry him, fulfilling Indra's promise. His heart wished and prayed for that. But he must be cautious. The planet, indeed the three worlds, were at stake.

He longed to know more about lovely Girikā. But diplomacy and decency demanded that he not press heavy issues on a convalescing queen, who was hosting him in her palace. So, he ventured a light-hearted observation that it was unusual for a queen to sit alone on a mountain.

She laughed. "You are a Kuru prince, and you spent years alone in the deep forest." Her voice turned grave. "I went to Mount Kolā-hala because I am mourning my dear father, the king. He recently left this world. I wanted to be alone to deal with my grief."

Vasu's attempt at clever banter had ended in disaster. He tried to undo the damage. "I'm truly sorry you lost your father. Be so kind as to accept my sincere condolences. Had I known, I would never have spoken as I did. Please forgive me."

His words pleased her. She thanked him and insisted that he need not apologize. Then, perhaps to help him avoid another clumsy query, she revealed that her mother, the queen, had also gone to the World Beyond.

"So," the young monarch concluded, "as the only child of my late parents, I rule alone. At least for now. But, if you permit me to ask, what brings you here to our country, so far from the Kuru lands?"

He then briefly explained how, having no kingdom, he renounced this world and aspired to Indra's world.

"I understand your decision, given the circumstances," Girikā said. "But, even in Indra's world, despite an extremely long lifespan, you will still be mortal. You will die, lose your celestial body, and fall again to Earth. Why aspire to that? Why not aspire to Viṣṇu's eternal world? Why pray to someone, and then seek a good life elsewhere? Forgive me, but I'm just curious."

Vasu stared, astonished. The young queen was actually preaching to him to accept Viṣṇu. An Asura would never do that. Asuras could be cunning and duplicitous. But they held it beneath their dignity and pride to feign devotion to their foe Viṣṇu, even for strategic gain. No, Queen Girikā was actually a Vaiṣṇavī, a devotee of Viṣṇu.

"Excuse me," she said, "but you're staring at me. Kindly reply to my questions."

Of course, he thought. Girikā is testing me, just as I was testing her! And with the same purpose.

He smiled broadly and apologized for staring. He knew he could tell Girikā the full truth, and he proceeded to do so. He revealed that Indra had personally come to see him, urging the prince to abandon his project of ascending to Indra's world. The prince should stay on Earth, to protect it.

"Lord Indra came to you!" she exclaimed. "That is extraordinary! I believe you, but why would Indra urge you to stay here to protect our planet? Protect it from what? From whom? Apart from a few recent, tragic incidents of beasts unnaturally killing forest sages, we have no problem on Earth. There is peace everywhere."

"Indeed, Queen Girikā, you react precisely as I did when Indra first told me to stay and protect this world. You ask the same questions."

"Indeed! So, how did Lord Indra change your mind? Was it by his personal grandeur and power? Or did he give you information that I and other monarchs do not presently possess?"

He glanced at Girikā, who remained grave. "Indra told me that the awful attacks on sages are but harbingers of far more terrible things to come. He further told me that I can reveal the whole truth only to my wife and children, and to those devoted to Viṣṇu."

"If I may ask," Girikā said, in what seemed like a disappointed tone, "who are your wife and children?"

"I'm sorry; I meant my future wife and children. I am not married."

"I see." She smiled. "You may safely consider me to be devoted to Viṣṇu."

Clearly, she was testing his trust in her. He did trust her, and told her the truth. "I do not wish to alarm you, but Asuras, taking birth as wild beasts, are attacking those sages devoted to Viṣṇu. The Asuras believe that by thus sabotaging Vaiṣṇava yajñas, they will weaken Viṣṇu, and ultimately destroy him. It pains me to say that, but I must tell you what Indra told me. Apart from that, Asuras are invading the Earth, taking birth in royal families. They will thus legally inherit powerful kingdoms, attack weaker realms, and gradually control this planet. They will then use Earth as a base from which to attack and subjugate the three worlds."

Girikā turned pale. It was her turn to silently stare. Vasu continued. "We must stop the Asuras here on Earth. Indra insisted that I would play a leading role in Earth's defense. He promised to make me a king — to be honest, the leading king." Here he stopped, studying Girikā's reaction.

She nodded silently, as if thinking deeply. Then she spoke. "Prince, I congratulate you on your great fortune. And you are absolutely sure that Indra told you that the Asuras — the Asuras who inhabit higher realms — are invading this Earth?"

"I am absolutely sure. There is no mistake."

"I see. This is most serious." Girikā lowered her head and closed her eyes in deep concentration. "Most serious indeed." She looked up, with wide-open eyes. "And to counter this threat, you will rule a kingdom, and eventually become king of kings."

"Yes," Vasu said. "I am to use my kingdom as a base from which to protect the world."

Girikā's irrepressible smile returned. "So you, a presently homeless royal, are to be king of kings on this planet."

"I swear on my honor, it was not my idea."

Girikā stood up, and began to pace the garden in which they had been sitting. She stopped, turned to face him, and said, "Tell me, did Indra mention which kingdom will be yours?"

Prince Vasu stood up to face her. Girikā's eyes bore down on him. Deception, even diplomacy, would fail with brilliant Queen Girikā.

"Forgive me, noble lady. I speak only what Great Indra told me. I am to rule this righteous kingdom of Cedi."

Girikā nodded. "Well, well, I confess I suspected as much. So, if we are to be practical here, you can only rule this land of Cedi in one of two ways."

Vasu looked carefully at her. "What are those two ways?"

Girikā smiled, but spoke boldly, as a proud monarch. "Prince Vasu, you must either defeat me in battle..." She paused.

"Or else...?"

"Or else you must win my heart."

Vasu gave out a sigh of relief, and a broad smile lit up his face. "I assure you," he said with a bow, "that I will never attack you, or your realm. I cannot speak for your heart, but if I may speak plainly, I fear you are rapidly winning mine."

Her face glowed at these words. With a mischievous smile, she said, "You fear I am winning your heart? Come, prince, surely you do not fear me."

Her smile was contagious. His heart stirred. Their eyes locked. He said, "I do not fear you. I know in my heart that you are too just and kind to pose any danger to an honest prince who seeks only the good of the world, and your happiness."

"Well spoken," she said, in high spirits. Having each indirectly expressed a growing love for the other, and agreeing that they must know each other better, since their acquaintance was so new, they sat closer together and eagerly spoke on many topics — political, moral, spiritual, personal — and agreed on every one. His attachment to her steadily grew, and she made no effort to conceal her pleasure in his company. That gave him courage to reveal his delight in hers. Vasu deeply relished this private meeting with Girikā, beyond the bustle and ceremony of royal attendants, and curious citizens.

They were royalty of a similar age and culture, with very similar natures. This made everything easy and natural between them. But the queen had a few lingering doubts. She believed in his courage and power. She knew that Cedi was safe in his hands. But how could he defend the sages in faraway lands from mighty Asuras roaming the Earth as savage beasts?

Her question reminded him of Indra's promise of a swift crystal fighting aircraft that would give Vasu an immense advantage over his foes. When would that aircraft come? He thought of Indra, and silently begged him to reveal the aircraft.

At once, a bright light appeared in the sky, outshining the daylight. Vasu and Girikā gazed in wonder as the light approached them. As it grew larger, they saw it was a heavily armed, aerodynamic fortress, speeding silently toward them and then slowly descending into a nearby meadow.

Girikā and Vasu raced there together, spontaneously grasping each other's hand. In its final approach, the wafting aircraft gently floated onto the emerald-green grass. A crystal plank silently emerged from the hull, came down, and softly touched the green grass. Fearsome missile launchers protruded from the hull in all directions. The aircraft seemed to beckon them aboard.

Girikā stepped back, distrustful. Vasu said, "I'm sure Lord Indra sent this aircraft to protect the Earth. He kept his promise. It must be safe. You can wait here and I will board it to see."

"I am a queen," Girikā said. "I will go with you."

Side by side, they walked up the crystal plank into the airship, and found it richly furnished and bristling with weapons, with unimpeded views all around.

"How do you drive it?" Girikā asked.

"I have a hunch," Vasu said. He focused his mind on the craft and willed it to ascend. The plank retracted with a hush and the ship rose steadily into the air, till they saw beneath them all of Pearl River and the surrounding countryside.

Vasu and Girikā looked at each other and gasped in wonder.

Vasu looked down. "The city is designed in the shape of a lotus!"

"Yes, it is." The queen smiled.

"And the fields, the orchards, and forests beyond the city walls are so manicured and precise. Cedi must rival Hastinā-pura itself."

The queen laughed. "That may be going too far. But Cedi is indeed a magnificent realm. By the way," Girikā said anxiously, "I assume you are controlling the craft."

"I think so. It responds to my mind. Watch! I now will it to fly to the North."

Instantly the aircraft moved to the North, without a sound.

"I am impressed," Girikā said. "This is definitely a Deva aircraft. Make it fly us to that river park." She pointed to a large, lush park that bordered Pearl River. "I mean, please do that, kind prince."

"Yes, Your Majesty." Vasu smiled. The aircraft silently sped there and landed.

"Wonderful!" Girikā said. They happily alighted from the aircraft, laughing and praising Indra's marvelous gift. They sat together by the river like old friends.

"I have a thought," Vasu said.

"So do I," she said.

"You first." He smiled.

"All right. The world will ever be grateful to you and Indra for your protection. That is my thought. What is yours?"

He hesitated, glancing at her with inquiring eyes. She tilted her head charmingly, as if to say, go ahead and tell me.

"Forgive me for what may seem like inappropriate haste. But I know my heart, and I pray to Viṣṇu that I have rightly understood yours. I ask you to accept me, as my very soul accepts you."

Queen Girikā smiled. "Are you asking me to marry you?"

"Yes."

"Then, yes. I will. My soul accepts you as your soul has accepted me."

It was settled. They soon headed back to the palace to explain what must surprise and please many.

Vasu and Girikā soon married with royal pomp and ceremony. For their honeymoon, they traveled around the world in the crystal airship, gazing down on Earth, gazing up at limitless stars. Mindful to ever use the crystal airship to serve humanity, they scoured Earth's forests for deadly Asura beasts, and with unfailing missiles, sent many of them back to their Asura world. Even on their honeymoon, they rescued many of Viṣṇu's brāhmaṇas.

CHAPTER 9

"King Vasu and Queen Girikā are my heroes!" cried Satya-vatī. "I admire them so much!"

Parā-śara laughed with pleasure. "I'm glad you feel that way," he said. "Very glad indeed."

"But who could not love and admire them? Really!"

"I agree," the sage said. "There is more to tell about them, but perhaps you'd like to rest first, or have lunch."

"Oh, Parā-śara! I feel I've been resting all my life. Please rest if you like, and I will patiently wait. But my only wish now is to hear more about my King and Queen."

Parā-śara laughed affectionately. "I am not tired, I assure you. What would you like to hear about the rulers of Cedi?"

"We know," Satya-vatī said, "that Vasu and Girikā have five excellent sons."

"Yes, they do. And with Indra's favor, Vasu became so powerful that he was able to give each son his own kingdom."

"What a blessed life the royal couple have lived, O sage, a life free of suffering. I am so grateful to you for kindly showing me all this. But I keep wondering why. Why do you tell me these things? I am an insignificant fisherman's daughter."

"That is a reasonable question," the sage said. "I knew you would ask, and the time has come to give you the answer."

Satya-vatī sat up straight, hardly breathing, fixed on his every word and tone.

"Kind maiden," the sage began, "you just said that the king and queen have enjoyed a blessed life, indeed, a life free of suffering."

"Yes," Satya-vatī said anxiously.

"In fact, though the world knows nothing of it, the life of King Vasu and Queen Girikā has not been entirely free of suffering. One great loss has given them much pain — the loss of their only daughter."

"Their daughter? But the emperor had no daughter."

"That is precisely what the world thinks," Parā-śara said. "You may know that King Vasu's middle son is Matsya."

"Yes, he is said to be most charming," Satya said. "Of the five Cedi princes, I've always thought that I would like Matsya best."

"Yes, he is charming, Satya. And so is his twin sister, though the world does not know she exists."

"Prince Matsya has a twin sister? Please, Parā-śara! Do not keep me in suspense."

"Forgive me, I will tell you everything."

Satya-vatī meditated deeply as Parā-śara revealed the following. Years ago, a few months before Queen Girikā was to give birth to a boy to be named Matsya, a mysterious brāhmaṇa couple appeared in the royal palace. No one knew how they entered. The couple wore robes with hoods that concealed their features. In tones so commanding that none dared disobey, they insisted on speaking in private with the royal couple. They were granted an audience.

Once alone with the king and queen, the sage couple lowered their hoods and revealed themselves to be the lords of the Deva realm, Indra and his wife Śacī. Vasu took the hand of Girikā, who froze in astonishment, and they bowed together to the Deva couple.

Vasu and Girikā, who overcame her shock, graciously welcomed their celestial visitors, thanked them for their visit, and begged to know how they might serve their guests. Lovely Śacī smiled and said, "Before all that, Girikā, please tell me how your pregnancy goes. How are you, dear queen?"

Awed by Śacī's kindness and beauty, Girikā said, "I am very well, thank you. I can hardly express how honored I am by your visit."

Śacī nodded, turned to her husband, and said, "Indra, it is best that you explain the purpose of our visit."

At Vasu's bidding, Indra and Śacī sat on elevated seats. Vasu and Girikā sat nearby. Indra began. "First, we thank you both for your excellent, faithful service. In fact, Vasu, seeing your strength and determination, the Asuras have chosen to simply wait until you are gone."

"Please explain," Vasu said.

Indra wasted no time. "As we know, Earth is martya-loka, the mortal world, a place where life is short, at least from the Deva or Asura point of view. So, the Asuras will just wait until your reign ends, and that of your sons. Then, in the third generation, they will attack with greater force than this world can imagine."

Girikā gasped. Vasu said, "Lord Indra, surely my grandsons will be worthy descendants of our line."

Śacī shook her head sadly. "There is a mighty Asura named Vipra-citti, eldest son of Danu. Counting you as the first generation of resistance against the Asuras, Vipra-citti will come in the third generation, bringing countless Asura legions with him. And in the fourth generation, his most deadly protégé, Kāla-nemi, will appear. One will inherit, and one will usurp, great kingdoms."

"Will the Devas come to protect this world?" Vasu asked.

"If we Devas come to Earth," Indra said, "we might not defeat the Asuras, and the battle alone would destroy this world. Also, if we come here directly, we will leave our own planets unprotected. Yet if the Asuras take the Earth, they will again attack the Devas, with renewed strength. So, you see our problem."

Vasu and Girikā nodded gravely. Girikā said, "So, what can be done? What can we do?"

Indra glanced at Śacī, who was no less somber. Indra spoke. "Vasu, you will continue to protect Earth, as you have done so well. Your sons will follow you. But Asura power will increase beyond what their sons can handle. Thus, an Avatāra is coming to help us. He is not Viṣṇu himself, but he will help greatly."

"An Avatāra is coming! Can it be true?" Girikā said.

"Yes," Śacī said. "He will take birth from a human mother, yet wield superhuman power."

"We rejoice at this news," Vasu said. "And we thank you from our hearts for the honor of this visit. Apart from our regular duties, is there anything more that Girikā and I can do?"

"There is one thing," Śacī said quietly. "You must be prepared to sacrifice something most dear to you."

Girikā turned pale. Vasu's face tightened, as if he were bracing himself. "My lords," he said, "what is that sacrifice?"

Śacī looked at Girikā and said, "Dear lady, you carry two souls in your womb. Twins. A boy and a girl. When they are born, you must give up the girl, your only daughter. In beauty and character, she will surpass all other girls. She will have a brilliant mind, and you will love her with all your heart, yet you must send her away the day she is born."

"Send her away?" Girikā said, still pale. "But why?"

"She has been chosen to give birth to an Avatāra, the first who will descend to oppose the Asura invasion. You, Vasu, are Earth's most powerful king. The Asuras watch you closely in ways you cannot detect. They sense an Avatāra is coming, and they will not hesitate to kill your daughter to prevent him from coming. I grieve for you," Śacī said, "but for your daughter's sake, and the world's sake, the child must be hidden. Send her away in absolute secrecy. Announce the birth of a son. Have a trusted aide take her far from the capital and entrust her to a decent couple, who will never be suspected of raising a princess, and who will never suspect it themselves. That couple cannot know your daughter's true identity. They might reveal it under pressure or torture, or give in to a large bribe. Indra and I will watch over her. No harm will come to her from any human being."

"You mean…" Girikā choked on her tears. "…you mean that if the Asuras find her, she will come to harm?"

"Yes," Śacī said softly. "More than harm. The Asuras will stop at nothing to eliminate your daughter. They must not find her. Place her where no one could ever suspect or imagine a princess would live. I'm so sorry, but as you know, we too are fighting against the Asuras. We all do what we must to protect those we love."

Śacī, queen of the Devas, wiped a tear from her eye. "We deeply regret this, but you must protect your daughter. Earth, and perhaps the three worlds, depend on it. You have our love and blessings."

With that, Indra and Śacī vanished from view. And all took place as they foretold. The twins took birth, and a trusted minister, well disguised, took the infant girl to a humble couple that led a fishing village on the bank of sacred Yamunā, far north of the capital. The couple was known to be of good character. They had repeatedly failed to produce a child, and this was the sorrow of their lives. They eagerly agreed to love this child as their own. They would raise the young girl with love and care. In their village lived good, simple folk who followed their leader and asked no questions. The couple would tell their people that relatives far down the river were unable to raise their daughter. The infant girl was to be raised as the natural daughter of the fishing couple. No one in the village, on pain of severe punishment, was ever to mention, even in private, that the child was adopted. The rule was followed strictly.

With grieving hearts, King Vasu and Queen Girikā received regular reports on their child from agents disguised as travelers. They never mentioned the child to others, not even their children. They occasionally flew over the village in their crystal aircraft. Deva-loka sent assurances that Indra and Śacī were watching over the child. The Asuras never discovered the secret, and the Cedi princess grew up to be a beautiful young lady.

The girl herself never suspected her true identity. She loved her adoptive parents, but she felt trapped, as if she didn't belong in that fishing village. Indeed, the most noble royal blood flowed through her. She even wondered why she didn't look like her parents. But she never imagined that she was an emperor's daughter, destined to give birth to an Avatāra.

"And that princess..." Satya gasped, "O sage, can you tell me who that princess is?"

"Of course. She sits in front of me. Her name is Satya-vatī."

CHAPTER 10

Satya-vatī sat stone silent. Parā-śara respected her silence and said nothing. Suddenly, she burst into tears, shaking with emotion. Parā-śara offered his support with earnest glances. After some time, her choking tears subsided.

"I'm sorry," she said, gasping for breath and wiping her eyes with her hands and cloth. He insisted that she need not apologize for anything.

After several more breathless minutes, she faced him with urgent questions in her eyes.

"I am here for you," he said quietly, "if there is anything that I can do."

She slightly bowed her head to thank him, and held up a hand to ask for a little more time. Finally, she was ready. Closing her eyes, she said, "Why didn't they tell me? I would have kept the secret."

Parā-śara breathed deeply, and said softly, "Your parents thought only of protecting you. They thought this was best. They could not know how strong and wise you are."

Satya-vatī nodded. Parā-śara saw that she understood but did not yet agree. He continued. "They knew the role you would play and did not wish to burden a child with that knowledge. They struggled with their decision. You were never out of their thoughts, but they thought it best to let you have a relatively carefree childhood, as long as possible. They also arranged for the brāhmaṇas across the river to invite you to study. Your parents arranged that."

"Yes, and that made all the difference. I did have loving parents, however simple they are, and I was well educated. I've had a good life. And I do not blame my birth parents. But was it really best to keep me in ignorance for so long? For years, even with my studies, I felt my life had no purpose. If I had known…"

"Satya, your parents truly feared for your life, and for the world. They acted with love. Why do you think the emperor of the world, and his queen, came to your little fishing village? It was to see you, because they loved you."

These words affected her. Her parents must truly love her. Parā-śara continued. "Whether they acted with perfect wisdom or should have told you sooner, I cannot say. And I will respect your feelings on this. But I know they always acted out of love for you."

Satya-vatī sighed. "I don't wish to blame them. And it means so much to me that my parents came to our little village. It was to see me! I wish I could be absolutely certain that my birth parents truly loved me. If I could erase that doubt from my heart, I might not suffer."

"Satya, did you ever notice a guardian star that often passes over your village?"

"How did you know that?" she exclaimed. "Yes, there is a star that often passes overhead at night, but only when I'm alone, and always on my birthday. That guardian star almost hovers above me, as if watching over me. I never told a soul about it. My parents would say I was dreaming or mad. I told no one."

Parā-śara smiled. "It is not a star, but it is two guardian angels — your own parents, Vasu and Girikā, watching over you in their crystal aircraft. They long to see you, to hold you in their arms. But to protect you in the only way they knew, they watched you from the sky, praying that Viṣṇu protect you."

Satya-vatī's body trembled with emotion and she wept with no power to stop. It took some time to compose herself. With tears still streaming down her face, she told Parā-śara that she believed her parents had always loved her.

In a moment, her expression changed dramatically, and her face turned white with a new anxiety. "Parā-śara, is it really me that will give birth to an Avatāra? That is terrifying!"

"Do you want to talk about that now?"

"Yes, of course. No, no, a little later. I'm not ready to talk about that. The thought makes me queasy. Please, tell me about the third generation. I am the second generation from my parents, and the next generation will really threaten the world. What is that third generation? Tell me quickly to take my mind off the Avatāra."

"Of course. Let's get straight to the point. Your brothers and so many other kings already have sons, who are the third generation."

Satya shivered with trepidation. "Surely you don't mean that the Asuras have come to my own family."

Parā-śara nodded slowly and said, "I'm sorry, Satya-vatī, but at least one very dangerous Asura has indeed come to your family."

"Oh God! What happened?"

"Your eldest and strongest brother is the celebrated Bṛhad-ratha, who now rules the powerful nation of Magadha. When your father retires, he will be senior among the five brothers who will jointly rule Cedi. Thus, he is clearly the head of your family's dynasty."

Here Parā-śara paused, pressed his lips together, then sighed with resignation. "Satya, do you remember I showed you the mighty Asura Vipra-citti?"

"Yes. He is their leader and the most frightening. He is leading the Asura invasion. Oh God, I dread what you are about to say."

"I'm sorry. But that most powerful Asura has already taken birth the first son and heir of your eldest brother, Bṛhad-ratha. The boy is known as Jarā-sandha, but he is absolutely Vipra-citti."

Satya gasped. "O Viṣṇu! Viṣṇu! Does Bṛhad-ratha know it?"

"Yes, he knows. But there is little he can do. By Dharma, his son will inherit the dynasty."

"So, when my eldest brother leaves this world…O Lord!"

"Yes, the Asura leader will inherit and rule the Cedi empire, the very dynasty that Indra empowered to save Earth from Asuras."

"That is awful, horrible."

"Yes, it is. That is why Indra himself, despite his pride, joined the other Devas in pleading for an Avatāra to descend."

Satya-vatī stood up, clasped her hands behind her back, and paced back and forth, her mind desperately calculating. "Couldn't Indra prevent Vipra-citti's birth as Jarā-sandha, if he knew about it?"

"Indeed, when Indra detected Vipra-citti in the womb of Bṛhad-ratha's wife, he tried to prevent the birth."

Satya stopped and faced the sage. "Oh, Parā-śara, how could Indra's power fail?"

"I will tell you. You have a right to know."

"Tell me, please, Parā-śara, but don't let me see it. I cannot bear to watch the most powerful Asura entering my own family."

Parā-śara stood up. "Of course. I will be brief. Let us walk a bit in the shade of the forest." Satya gratefully agreed. The sage took a few steps, and began speaking.

"Vipra-citti knew that Indra chose your father, Vasu, to lead the resistance against the Asura invasion. Rather than confront your father and Indra directly, he engaged his own mercenary brāhmaṇas in performing yajñas that increased his power. When he believed his power sufficient to confront Indra, he took birth in your family. He studied your brothers closely and then chose Bṛhad-ratha to be his father."

"Why Bṛhad-ratha?" Satya-vatī asked quietly.

"As the first born, Bṛhad-ratha is the most powerful of your brothers, politically and militarily. Thus, the so-called Jarā-sandha will inherit the leadership of your family dynasty. Since he has not violated Dharma, and, indeed, since Dharma itself protects his right of inheritance, his father cannot stop him. Also, Bṛhad-ratha is not a native of Magadha. The citizens follow him, but will naturally be more inclined, in case of a family dispute, to give their sympathy to one of their own."

"Such as Prince Jarā-sandha."

"Exactly."

They kept walking. Satya sighed but continued her strategic analysis. It came naturally to her. "When did Indra discover Vipra-citti's plan?"

"Almost as soon as Vipra-citti entered your sister-in-law's womb. Of course, he could not allow this, and so he attacked the embryo, without harming the mother."

"And what happened?" Satya asked anxiously.

"Vipra-citti realized he was under attack and fought back. With his Vajra bolt, Indra succeeded in bifurcating the embryo, but he could not kill it. Vipra-citti's powers are truly prodigious. Though Indra rendered the Asura's body unworkable, Vipra-citti kept his divided body alive, to Indra's great frustration."

"What happened then?" Satya-vatī asked.

"Well, as you can imagine, the birth of two living, and perfectly symmetrical, halves of a baby's body shocked the mother nearly to death. Deeply traumatized and not realizing the halves were living, she ordered a servant to cast them into the deep forest."

"And did the servant do that?"

"Yes, she did. What Indra could not foresee was that a powerful Asura yoginī named Jarā was monitoring the birth and rushed to the discarded, still-living halves of Vipra-citti's body."

"I see," Satya said, as they stopped and sat together on a soft patch of green grass, deep in the forest. "The Asuras planned this well. So, what did the Asura yoginī Jarā do then?"

"With her Asura power, she fused the two body halves together, without a trace of separation; Vipra-citti's body was made whole. Disguised as a respectable lady of the country, Jarā then clasped the healthy babe to her breast and hurried to the Magadha capital. She presented the baby to the king and queen, who showered her with gifts and gratitude. After believing they had lost their child, the royal couple became all the more attached to him upon his miraculous return."

"I see," Satya-vatı said, amazed by the story. "But Indra must have informed Bṛhad-ratha, and our father, Vasu, about the child's real identity."

"Yes, Indra informed them both, but it was too late. News of the child's miraculous recovery had already spread throughout the city and kingdom. All of Magadha saw the child as a gift of the Devas, though the truth was exactly the opposite. Bṛhad-ratha could not reveal his son's identity, without causing widespread panic. In the meantime, the citizens grew firmly attached to the boy. They pressured the king to declare a state holiday with grand festivities to celebrate his son's return. The king knew he could not kill his own son when Indra had failed to kill him. And had the king tried to disinherit his son, the people would have revolted. After all, Jarā-sandha was born, miraculously, in Magadha. Bṛhad-ratha and his wife are from Cedi."

Satya-vatī gasped. "Oh heaven, what a fiasco!"

"Yes, and it gets worse. In yet another dark twist, because the Asura Jarā joined the baby's two halves, she became a national hero in Magadha, a country meant to protect the Earth from Asuras. In fact, it was the Magadha people who began calling the child Jarā-sandha, 'joined by Jarā,' and the name stuck."

"How odious!" Satya-vatī said. "The Asura commander Vipra-citti is now living on Earth as my own dear nephew."

"Yes. And within your lifetime, he will inherit the Cedi dynasty. That, Satya-vatī, is the problem that we and all the world face."

Satya-vatī and Parā-śara now walked along the river, away from the brāhmaṇa village. Satya drew strength from goddess Yamunā, and concentrated on her duty to Viṣṇu and the Devas.

She turned to Parā-śara. "Kindly tell me, who is the Avatāra that is to become my child?"

"His official name will be Vyāsa. He will prepare the world for Viṣṇu, his master. You see, even Avatāras serve Viṣṇu."

"But how will Vyāsa prepare the world for Viṣṇu? What will he do?"

"Well, among other things, he is a literary figure."

"A literary figure? Parā-śara, how will literature stop the Asuras? Are you joking with me?"

"Satya, I said among other things, he is literary. And you have to see what I mean by literary."

"Forgive me. Please explain. I'm just nervous about all this."

"Of course. You have good reason to be. Satya-vatī, surely you have heard of the Veda, the Book of Knowledge."

"Yes, of course. Everyone has heard of it. And the brāhmaṇas of Kalpi study it daily. My parents — I mean my foster parents — never talk about it. They say it's for brāhmaṇas, not fishing folk."

"I see. Anyway, you undoubtedly heard from the sages that the Veda teaches us Law, and duty — Dharma. But the Veda is so vast, so complex, that even brāhmaṇas now struggle to understand it."

"Yes, the sages told me the knowledge is fading. Each generation understands less of the Veda. I didn't know what they meant."

"That is why," Parā-śara said, "Avatāra Vyāsa has, among other tasks, a literary job to perform. He will save the true understanding of Veda. People are losing their grasp of Dharma and thus losing their power to fight evil. Vyāsa will teach the world what they have forgotten. The world will then defend itself, by defending Dharma. When protected, the Law protects. When attacked, it attacks in a most devastating way. Moreover, Vyāsa will chronicle the story of Viṣṇu so powerfully that present and future generations will rally to his side, and resist the Asuras. And in other ways, Vyāsa will play a key role in the struggle against the Asuras. The Asuras will be desperate to stop him, and the easiest way to do that is to stop him from ever taking birth."

Satya-vatī sat up straight as a warrior, feeling royal blood run through her veins. "I see," she said. "If people do not know Law, they violate it. This violation renders them weak before the Asuras. Through his teachings, Avatāra Vyāsa will teach humanity, now and in the future, the real meaning of the Veda, the universal Law. With this knowledge, people of Earth will happily support Viṣṇu, who will gladly reciprocate by saving their planet."

"Brilliant!" cried Parā-śara. "I see why you were chosen for this sacred task. You are a wise soul."

"Oh, I only repeat what I have heard from the wise. I have done nothing yet. But I want to help. What else will Avatāra Vyāsa do? You said he had many tasks."

"Vyāsa will personally prepare the way for Viṣṇu by protecting the Earth until his master appears. Vyāsa will then chronicle all of Viṣṇu's deeds. And when Viṣṇu has gone, countless generations to come will learn of these events through Vyāsa's words. They will guide many souls for thousands of years."

"And this same Vyāsa will be my son. It seems like a dream."

"Like a dream, but very real," Parā-śara said.

His words brought Satya-vatī back to anxious consideration of practical details. "I have no idea," she said nervously, "exactly how Avatāras are born. Will he just...enter...I mean will I just suddenly be...pregnant?"

"Not exactly. There will be a father who will...beget Vyāsa...in the conventional sense of begetting."

Satya-vatī turned white. "And who is that father? I can't just have a child with someone I don't even know or love, and certainly not with a man who is not my husband."

"Satya-vatī," Parā-śara said softly, "I understand how you feel. I know how difficult this is for you, to hear so many heavy things at once. Now, it is my sacred duty to tell you something else that I know will strike you as strange, and perhaps awful. I assure you this was not my idea. But...it seems that I am to be the father. This sacred duty was given to me. Please believe that."

Nothing had prepared Satya-vatī for this revelation and it thus fell upon her with dizzying force. So deep was her reverence for the brāhmaṇas that despite her attraction, even her attachment, to Parā-śara, she could not think of him as anything but a holy sage. The father of her child? How could she overcome a veneration she had felt for sages since early childhood?

As her mind whirled, Satya-vatī blushed deeply. Realizing this, she blushed even more. She hardly knew where she was.

"I'm sorry," she stammered, "I didn't expect this. Forgive me, but are we supposed to marry? I intend no offense, but you must know that normally men propose marriage before they propose procreation. I'm sorry, you are a great sage, and I'm sure you are doing your duty, but I am not ready for this. Will we marry?"

"We will not. That is not the plan. I cannot stay on Earth."

Satya-vatī felt herself sinking into the Earth. Her mind reeled. Pale and trembling, she said, "Parā-śara, my parents! My step-parents! And the brāhmaṇas, and the world! What will they all think?"

"I understand," Parā-śara said. "I really do. I will simply say that the world will know nothing about this, not for generations. Also, after the divine child is born, your body will regain its virginity."

"That's fine!" Satya-vatī cried in great distress, "but how will the world not know? Everyone will see that I am with child, before and after his birth. My life will be ruined. Parā-śara, I thought you came to save me, not to destroy me."

"Satya-vatī, please hear the whole plan before you judge it."

"I'm sorry, brāhmaṇa, I'm sorry," she said, steadfastly shaking her head in refusal, as the rest of her body trembled.

"Satya-vatī, please listen. I beg you. The Avatāra will take birth in less than an hour after conception. At his birth, before your eyes, he will grow into a youth. He will bid you farewell and transfer himself to a secluded hermitage high in the great mountains. Great yogīs there will make sure the Asuras do not detect him. Vyāsa will gather his powers there and prepare his mission."

"So I will never see my own child again?"

"Not for several years. Satya-vatī, to save this world, to save the three worlds, we are called upon to do selfless service. You will not have the joy of raising the Avatāra. That would be too dangerous for you and your son. Your parents made a similar sacrifice."

"But my parents had other children. And they had each other. I am to do all this, to make this sacrifice, alone? Why me?"

"Because you are an extraordinary soul. You were chosen for your noble qualities, your devotion and strength. As the Avatāra's mother, you will be called upon in the future to play an important role in the battle against the Asuras."

"But you and I?" Satya-vatī said. "What will we do after our son is born?"

Parā-śara looked down. "Satya, I am a brāhmaṇa and you are a princess. You and I have…an affinity, but in the end, we have very different natures. One of us would be forced to adopt an unnatural existence. For the good of the world, with genuine affection for each other, our duty is just to bring an Avatāra into this world."

"And what is my future in this world, or should I simply end it all in the Yamunā? Perhaps I should let the dear goddess take me where she will, to another world."

"Satya, please. Viṣṇu will not forget you. He loves you as much as dear Yamunā. There is a plan. Believe me. Someday you will marry high royalty. You will live a happy life. You will know real love, I assure you. But that married life is not with me."

Satya-vatī breathed deeply, struggling to regain her composure. When she felt she had achieved sufficient self-control, she said, "Dear sage, when will I be able to reveal my royal birth? We know that no prince or king would ever marry a fisherman's daughter. You are a holy sage. Tell me the truth, I beg you."

"Satya-vatī, I swear you will be rewarded. Trust me. You will find the happiness you seek."

Satya-vatī slumped down, her mind racing, but going nowhere. Finally, she covered her face and wept. At last, she looked up and gasped, "Oh sage, I'm sorry, truly sorry. But you've told me more than I can bear — that all my life I lived by a false identity; that I am to beget a child out of wedlock, and with you, whom I revere as a holy sage! My mind is shattered. I cannot bear it. I cannot do what you ask. I beg you, sage, forgive me!"

Remembering, with heart in pain, the first time they met, Satya-vatī bowed to the sage and ran toward her boat. She hardly knew what she said to the elderly brāhmaṇas who greeted her as she raced to the riverbank. Confused and exhausted, she labored to row against the current toward her village. Her mind grew feverish with agitation. She had refused a divine mandate. She had rejected Parā-śara's plea. She refused a divine entreaty to help her planet.

Satya-vatī's long cherished hopes for a better life seemed to sink into the river. Did Yamunā herself, dear goddess of the river, now reject her?

CHAPTER 11

As she approached her village, Satya-vatī was in no condition to speak with those whom she now knew to be foster parents. With weak arms, she rowed past the village, and went to her favorite hiding place, a small, thickly wooded island in a wide stretch of the Yamunā, just beyond a sharp bend, out of view of her village. No one else ever went there, and she was not fit to answer the many questions her parents were sure to ask.

Parā-śara's flurry of revelations had stunned, exhausted, and finally overwhelmed her. Now, in a hidden inlet of her private island, tucked out of view even of passing boats, Satya-vatī sat limp, bobbing in her boat, as gentle waves lapped the hull.

She could not have felt more separated from the loving couple that raised her than she did now. They had concealed from her the half-truth they knew, that they adopted her because her real parents could not raise her. Now Satya must hide from them the full truth of her identity.

How their roles had reversed! All her life, they knew more than she did about her origin. Now, she knew more. And she would conceal her superior knowledge from them, just as they had concealed theirs from her. The irony was striking, but held little interest for her in her present state.

Yet, there was some good in this. She would no longer be vexed by vague, hazy dissatisfactions, by inscrutable feelings of not truly belonging. But she had no time to celebrate this good, because an even more absurd irony now forced itself upon her. Having just learned that she was a princess from the most noble royal line, she had celebrated the grand revelation by refusing, and thus failing, to act with noble selflessness.

Her father and mother acted boldly for the world's good. But they were in love. They had each other. Parā-śara was clearly not in love with her, though he treated her with genuine respect and affection.

What were her feelings for Parā-śara? He himself described it. They had "genuine affection for each other." His words gave her comfort. He was right. They were not deeply in love. Still, genuine affection between two souls was something, something to be remembered with pleasure and gratitude. Indeed, to gain such affection from such an exalted sage could not but gratify her. However Satya might strive to free herself from pride, Parā-śara's affection for her must swell her heart. But there was no future between them. She must keep her feelings within bounds, as he did.

She had refused to help him save the world. Now, to ward off waves of guilt, she told herself that great souls like Parā-śara and Indra, not to speak of most powerful Viṣṇu, could easily find another girl, a far better girl, to become the Avatāra's mother.

She must think no more about it. She thought of her brothers, the Cedi princes. They were good souls, but not as powerful as their father. She thought with painful compassion of her eldest brother, Bṛhad-ratha, who must raise as his own son, and appear to love, his greatest enemy — indeed, Earth's greatest enemy. Jarā-sandha, knowing his true identity and mission, must himself cynically feign affection for his father. And Bṛhad-ratha's wife, Satya's sister-in-law — she must know her son's identity! How Satya longed to comfort her eldest brother and sister-in-law. How she yearned to help them. Yet they did not even know she existed. And she had rejected her chance to render practical aid to them, to the cause of Dharma, indeed, the cause of Viṣṇu. How these thoughts tormented her!

The sun was now sinking into the western waters. Creature cries broke the dusk stillness. She must return to her village and do her best to seem normal. Well, normal was impossible, but she would do all she could not to alarm her family.

Satya thought she was behaving almost as usual as she docked her boat at the village. But her mother took one look at her and cried out to the Devas. Satya touched her own face and realized that tears were still flowing down her cheeks.

Her father came running, looked at Satya, and shook his head, reaching his hands to the sky. He prayed to the Devas to reveal what he had done wrong. Satya-vatī had no strength to dodge their predictable questions, nor fend off their equally predictable entreaties. So she hugged them both, and insisted she was fine, but exhausted, and just needed rest. She hurried to her cottage (she had long ago insisted on having her own cottage), only to lie sleepless, imploring Viṣṇu to grant her strength and wisdom, since at the moment she felt she had neither.

The next day's sun rose upon a still-bewildered Satya-vatī. The courageous example of her birth parents, and her own heart, troubled her. She refused Parā-śara's proposal, which he claimed came from high authority. If she persisted in her refusal, what would she do with her life?

No one could imagine that she was a princess whose father ruled the world. Satya-vatī could not tell anyone the truth without causing havoc to those she loved most. Parā-śara had promised she would be rewarded for her sacrifice, if she would only accept it. She now assumed that her refusal would cancel the rewards that would come with her acceptance.

So, I refuse to bring the Avatāra, she thought. That means I continue to suffer, increasingly, in this village, and my life is meaningless. For the Avatāra's sake, my parents gave up their only daughter, a daughter they truly love, and I now render their painful sacrifice, and my own, meaningless. Asuras threaten the world, and I gamble the fate of millions on my assumption that some other girl will do the job.

Deeply troubled, Satya-vatī boarded her boat and let it drift on the gentle, rocking currents of Yamunā. She implored the river goddess to give her wisdom and courage.

On gentle waves, the goddess carried her slowly toward the brāhmaṇa village. Was Heaven bringing her back to Parā-śara? She saw sages bathing in the river, tending sacred fires, reciting ageless mantras.

"Please!" Satya cried aloud to Yamunā. "Sweet goddess of the river, I can't do it! Forgive me, I beg you. I have always loved you since earliest childhood. Now I entreat you, intercede on my behalf, convince the great ones to choose another girl."

But the river brought her closer to the brāhmaṇa shore. All her life she had served these sages. And dear Parā-śara was revered by all the sages that she revered. She had refused him. What if the world really depended on her? What if Viṣṇu himself was testing her devotion?

As she fretted, a deafening roar shattered the still air, shaking Satya's heart. She froze and looked. Huge tigers moved toward the sages. The beasts roared with unbearable ferocity, exceeding all that is natural to Earth. The elderly sages cried out the alarm.

"Oh God, the Asuras have come!" Satya gasped, as the beasts closed in on the sages. "Oh, Parā-śara!" she wailed silently. "O Heaven protect them! Protect the sages!"

Suddenly, a blazing light raced across the river. She looked up. Below the clouds, King Vasu in his crystal aircraft came flying at startling speed. Satya-vatī trembled with joy. Her own father, mighty Vasu, would answer her prayer.

Indeed, the king of kings lit up the sky with flashing weapons. His fiery missiles struck the Asura beasts with pitiless precision. Proud, demonic roars turned into death shrieks.

Loving, ecstatic pride in her father filled Satya's heart. "He is truly the king of kings," she whispered to herself.

Then all was silence. The aircraft vanished as quickly as it appeared. Satya gazed at the empty sky in wonder, but just for a moment. She saw a wounded sage on the beach. She rushed her boat to the shore, frantic to help, and to see if Parā-śara were still alive.

An elderly brāhmaṇa lay dying on the sand. Satya had always loved him as a grandfather, and he had fully returned her love. She rushed to him and did all she could to bring comfort to his last moments on Earth. As he passed on, his head cradled in her hands, she felt a righteous rage she had never felt before. With frightening resolve, she swore to Viṣṇu himself that she would do whatever was needed to stop the Asura invasion. She knew what those words meant.

But was Parā-śara alive? She had been hidden since birth, she had endured an unnatural life, just to perform the one crucial act of bringing an Avatāra to the world. After all that, had the Asuras discovered and destroyed the plan at the last moment by killing Parā-śara?

By now, boatloads of fishermen, led by her father, arrived at the scene, knowingly risking their lives to help the sages. At that moment, her heart filled with love and respect for these simple, good people. The fishermen and sages mixed like never before. Both cried out in praise of King Vasu. Their words thrilled her, but there was no time to lose. Before her father could stop or question her, she ran to the woods in search of Parā-śara. Where was he? Perhaps he lost his faith in her and left the night before, or early that morning. This thought filled her heart with pain.

She climbed to higher ground, but as far as she could see, there was no trace of Parā-śara. A young fisherman her age came running and said, "Your father wants to see you at once. Satya, you have to come."

She complied, too shaken to argue. Her stepfather embraced her and said, "Satya, you must go home now. Please do not fight with me at a time like this. We have more than enough men here to take care of everything. If we need help, we'll send word to the ladies, I promise you."

She saw that it would be cruel to argue with him in these circumstances. The fishermen would take excellent care of the sages. And the horror of the attack, and Parā-śara's departure, left Satya-vatī devastated and drained. She offered affectionate, heartfelt words to the sages, returned to her boat, and pushed off. She had no intention of returning to the village to face endless questions and admonitions from her mother and the other ladies. She could return to her secluded isle to rest and grieve alone. But even that idea was soon drowned in a sea of misery. With no strength to row or steer in any direction, she slumped down in her boat and wept uncontrollably.

CHAPTER 12

Satya-vatī had never in her young life felt so spent in mind and spirit. After a life of boredom and frustration, she met a celebrated young sage who seemed to truly like her. He gave her life-changing revelations of her royal family. He invited her to play a key role in saving the world.

And here she was, drifting aimlessly, literally and figuratively, more alone than ever. She had not only lost Parā-śara, she could never think of her fishing family in the same way. For all their limitations, she had seen them as her real family. Now, even that was lost.

She could approach her royal family in Pearl River. But, having failed in her sacred mission to bring an Avatāra to the world, how would they receive her? They had given their lives for the very mission she rejected. They might even blame her for endangering the world. Were he to accept her, King Vasu would have to explain to all the citizens why he sent her away in the first place. That would be very difficult without revealing the Asura invasion and putting all the citizens in panic. No, she would not go to her birth family in a shameful state.

Eventually, the Asuras would attack, and the whole world would blame her. Even if the Devas did choose another girl, that girl would be hailed as a heroine. Satya-vatī would live in the world's memory as a symbol of failure of spirit.

The idea of returning to her old life as a fisherman's daughter depressed her exceedingly. She could no longer bear it. Perhaps she would simply let her boat drift on to another country. But that too was impossible. The heartless world would think the worst of a young lady traveling alone to a strange country.

Satya-vatī knew that some hopeless souls overcame misery by tying a stone to their ankle and sinking into a sacred river. But such an act would surely displease dear Yamunā. In short, Satya-vatī could find no comfort in life or death.

She wept bitterly; her body shook. Mindless of where the waters took her, she lost all sense of time. When she finally looked around, she found herself at the shore of her secret island. Perhaps she would deploy all she learned from the dear sages and fast in meditation till Viṣṇu took her from this suffering world. After all, she had nothing to live for.

Parā-śara emphatically promised her rewards in this world, including a loving marriage, if she would only help him. But she had refused. Now, she could not rationally expect those blessings that were to reward the fulfillment of a sacred task she refused to perform.

She respected her own body as a divine gift, and she would not harm it in a suicidal act. Yet she now had no reason to do anything but sit quietly on her special island, fix her mind on Viṣṇu, and await a better future life.

Then Viṣṇu spoke to her from within her heart, and gently helped her to understand that he had chosen her to perform a great service for this world. Satya felt joy and shame, joy that Viṣṇu had chosen her and shame that she had rejected her sacred mission. But it now seemed too late. Parā-śara was gone! With deep regret, and despair, Satya docked her boat and stepped onto her island. She walked with weak steps to a little meadow surrounded by flowering trees. There she sat, until a familiar voice called out to her, "Satya-vatī, I'm so glad to see you."

It was Parā-śara! A second chance! She tried to be calm and gracious, but she could not conceal her excitement and embarassment. She must reply to his kind greeting, but she struggled to find the words. She managed, "Dear sage, thank you for receiving me so kindly." She could say no more. She regretted having refused him before, and she was too nervous to renew the topic, much less reveal how her feelings had changed. She must depend on him to lead the conversation. He seemed willing to do so.

With concern and respect, he inquired about her thoughts and feelings. What did she think was best? What should they do? There was hope in his voice, hope they could together perform a sacred duty. And he clearly evinced genuine regard for her. Seeing that he did not blame or reject her, but rather seemed eager to renew their tie, Satya-vatī admired him more than ever. Now she could openly converse with him.

Each opened their heart to the other. And with remarkably few words, they agreed to act together to bring the Avatāra.

A fishing boat glided past the island. Satya and Parā-śara exchanged knowing glances. They must have greater seclusion, beyond the eyes of the world. Parā-śara smiled and raised his hand. Instantly a thick fog that was neither cold nor damp shrouded the island. Strong currents began to push away from the island. No boat could now see or approach them.

Satya knew the time was drawing near to bring the Avatāra. "I have some… concerns," she said softly. "May I ask you now?"

"Of course. Please, anything."

"The Asuras will not attack me in revenge?"

"No, they will not unnecessarily offend Dharma by attacking a woman. It would do them no good, only terrible harm."

"Will the Asuras attack my son?"

"They would like to, but our son will be safe. I will personally take him to the Himālaya. There, powerful sages will be with him."

"Thank you. Will I meet my real parents?"

"That is your decision. I only ask that you be discreet so that you do not put them or yourself in danger. I know you understand. You are a brilliant young lady with natural political instincts."

Satya-vatī lowered her head and thanked him, but did not say more.

"You must be concerned," he said, "about your future after your son and I go."

"Yes, I am deeply concerned," she said. "Now that I know my identity, how will I live in this village? What will I do?"

"Be hopeful. Viṣṇu will reward your selfless service to the world."

"Can you say more about that?"

"I will say this, Satya-vatī. You will find love and happiness. Trust me. A great king will marry you. You will love each other dearly."

Satya looked into Parā-śara's eyes. She found no lust there, no pride, only an unbreakable determination to help other souls and to protect the world. And she saw in his eyes genuine affection for her. Confident of his purity, and his knowledge of her future, she said, "Perhaps the time has come to bring the Avatāra."

He nodded. "Yes, the time has come. Viṣṇu has spoken to you from within your heart."

Fully realizing now the extraordinary gravity of her task, she asked, "Parā-śara, where shall I fix my consciousness? What should my thoughts be?"

"We must both remember," he said, "that you and I are eternal spiritual beings, engaging material bodies in sacred service. We must fix our minds in our own true self, and the true self of the other. Then we must see our pure selves within the mind of Viṣṇu. We will then envision the Avatāra as an expansion of Viṣṇu's infinite mind."

"And our pure awareness of him," Satya-vatī said, "will draw him to us. Isn't that true?"

"Yes, it is true." Parā-śara smiled. "You understand perfectly. Satya-vatī, you have been wisely chosen."

Satya-vatī and Parā-śara sat together in meditation. Within their hearts, they saw their eternal, luminous selves. And each saw the other's eternal being. Their true selves were personal, beautiful. The bodily identity was but a shadow of the true self. In this pure state of awareness, Satya-vatī experienced freedom from fear, attachment and aversion, longing and lamentation. It was a state of exquisite, absolute joy, beyond anything she had imagined possible.

Satya opened her eyes. Simply by a glance, an expression, Parā-śara guided her in the act of begetting. She transcended her self and saw within her heart the infinite Self of Viṣṇu. At her instant of maximum clarity, the act of conception took place. Within moments, Satya's abdomen swelled with the Avatāra's presence. She felt no pain. Minutes later, to Satya-vatī's utter amazement, the Avatāra came into this world, glowing with his own luster. His features were fine, his expression precociously cognizant, yet he was a newborn child. Parā-śara placed the celestial babe in his mother's arms, and she adored him.

Parā-śara then held out his hand and a soft cotton blanket appeared on the pliant meadow grass. He took the babe in his arms and placed it on the cloth. Before his parents' eyes, the baby quickly grew. Within minutes, the glowing child stood up gracefully as a handsome young boy. He joined his palms in veneration and bowed to his father and mother.

Parā-śara nudged the astonished mother, and she ran to embrace her child. Parā-śara followed her. Holding the child to her breast, Satya-vatī asked the father, "What shall we call him? What is he meant to be called?"

Nodding to the child, Parā-śara said, "This boy was born on an island, dvīpa. So, we shall call him Dvaipāyana, the Island-born. But for now, we alone shall know his name. The world will call him Vyāsa, the arranger of the Veda."

Still embracing the boy, Satya-vatī said through her tears, "Your father has given you a beautiful name. You are Dvaipāyana."

The child smiled and bowed to his parents. He spoke in a clear voice. "Thank you. I will honor and love you as my parents. But the world must not know of me yet. Forgive me, Mother, but I must go to the Himālaya. As you know, I have an urgent mission."

"I know," Satya-vatī said anxiously. "But what will you do there?"

"I will meditate and awaken all my powers. Then I shall begin my work before the Asuras grow too strong. I will arrange and compose the sacred knowledge, for it will protect the people of Earth. Mother, we shall meet again, I promise you. And if ever you truly need me, you need only think of me and I will come at once. I promise you this."

Satya-vatī stared in wonder at Avatāra Dvaipāyana. He inhabited the body of a child, but he spoke with the assurance of a most senior sage.

"Mother," he said, "you have undergone a threefold sacrifice. You were separated at birth from your real parents. Now, both my father and I must depart. You will be blessed more than you can imagine for your sacrifice."

"Are you sure you'll be safe?" Satya-vatī asked.

"Yes. Please don't worry. I regret that I am to leave. But I must perform the duty for which I came to this world."

"I understand," she said. "Your father explained everything."

The glowing child glanced at Parā-śara, who nodded and said, "Dear Satya-vatī, the time has come. We must leave. I will be ever grateful to you for all you have done. I shall never forget you."

Satya-vatī beckoned him to a place where her son could not hear, and asked him, "How can I live here now in this village? Oh sage, what will I do?"

Parā-śara grasped her hand and said, "I promise you that a great man will love you, and you shall love him. Believe me, Satya, I beg you."

"I do believe you," she said, and they returned to the Avatāra child. Parā-śara took the child's hand. They bowed to Satya-vatī and vanished before her eyes. Astonished, hopeful, and sad, she waved to them though they had gone.

The fog vanished with them, along with the strong river currents. The sun shone on a gently moving river. Satya-vatī sat for some time, lost in thoughts and memories. Although Parā-śara and her son had protected her from all the pain and exhaustion of childbirth, Satya-vatī's aching heart weakened her, and she had just enough strength to get into her boat. A wind carried her safely back to the fishing village.

At the little dock, she sat resting in her boat, too weak to move. Her parents found her there. Satya did not realize that a soft light emanated from her, for she had been touched by the Avatāra.

"What happened?" her mother asked with tender concern. "Is it the shock of the horrible beasts?"

"Yes," she said, dreading further conversation. "Please don't worry. That poor sage will surely go to the World Beyond. I will be all right."

"My dear daughter!" cried her mother. "You look different. Father, do you see it?"

"She looks the same to me," Dāśa-rāja said. "We've all been through an ordeal. We're all shaken."

"Never mind," her mother said. "She just seemed to glow for a moment, but it was my imagination."

With her foster parents' help, Satya-vatī returned to her cottage. After that day, she was unable to perform her old duties. She took to wandering in the forest and drifting on the river. She went less often to the brāhmaṇa village, for memories of Parā-śara, and of the Asura attack, still pained her.

She wandered in the deep woods. Her stepparents watched and worried but could do nothing. She realized more than ever the truth of Parā-śara's words. Her true nature was that of a princess, not a sage. This realization eased her pain at the loss of Parā-śara.

Seeing their only child hopeless and depressed, Dāśa-rāja and his wife grew desperate to help her, to do anything that might restore the girl's will to live. They approached her one day and actually suggested that she visit the Cedi capital, Pearl River, to see the king of kings.

"Dear child," her father said, "King Vasu just returned from a victorious campaign, and will stay in his capital for some time. You always wanted to visit Pearl River and see the king."

"Yes," her mother added. "Oh Satya, it's what you always wanted. Surely, a trip to the great capital will lift your spirits."

Since learning her real identity, Satya-vatī had given up the idea of visiting the capital. She knew that her real parents would be unable to acknowledge her, and this would be more painful than anything. She did not blame them. How could they explain why they sent their only daughter away? No doubt, Asura spies lived in the Cedi capital, and perhaps had infiltrated the government. Were Emperor Vasu to reveal that Asuras had invaded the world, the Asura agents themselves would spread panic among the population, and thus try to destabilize governments loyal to the Devas. Painful as it was, she concluded that her birth parents could not in good faith reveal her identity to the world. But they might admit it within the tight family circle. They might acknowledge her, love her, and that would change everything. Indeed, they would be proud of her for doing her duty, and bringing an Avatāra into the world. And, surely, they would treat her with great compassion, knowing the sacrifices she had made.

Thus reflecting, Satya concluded that the idea of going to Pearl River might not be as absurd as it first seemed. She would go. In fact, she was now determined to go. She tried hard to put out of her mind the danger that her family might not acknowledge her. They might not believe her. What proof did she have that she was truly their daughter? They might suspect her of being an Asura agent!

But that fear could not stop her! She would go. She *must* go. She had nothing else to do, while she waited anxiously for Parā-śara's promise of future happiness to come true.

CHAPTER 13

The fisher king and his wife would never allow their child to travel alone to Pearl River. They arranged a trustworthy fishing couple to accompany her down to the capital. Satya did insist that she and her chaperones travel in separate boats. This was a practical necessity: three passengers with their luggage would never fit in Satya's boat or theirs.

Satya had another motive. Her chaperones were good, kind people, but low in their manners, speech, and dress. If she entered the great capital with them, she would be marked at once as a low-class girl. It was too embarrassing. Satya thus insisted on taking her own boat and devised a plan to escape from her older companions.

As she left her village for the first time, Satya's excitement, her joyous sense of escape, mingled with sadness and guilt. She was leaving the only parents she had ever known. They stood on the shore waving and touching their hearts as she boarded her boat. She waved and touched her heart, but she could not feel what she imagined they felt. A sense of guilt pained her for she felt what they would feel if they knew how eagerly she left what for them was the whole world.

Satya did feel gratitude — she loved her adoptive parents — but her life with them was hopeless. Now that she had the luxury of hope of a future, she could be generous and regret all the harsh words she had spoken to them since she was old enough to realize where she was and where she longed to be. So she waved to them and touched her heart, with earnest prayers and wishes for their happiness without her, for her life there was over.

As the river goddess Yamunā carried her south, and the village vanished from view, Satya thought of Dvaipāyana, her beautiful, glowing child that needed no mother. She smiled in wonder through the tears she wept at his perpetual absence.

Floating on Yamunā's currents past farms and forests, waving to children at play on the shore, bowing to sages meditating on the shore, Satya made her way toward a family that did not know her, would not recognize her, and could not imagine she would appear among them.

Even if she told them her identity, they would have to conceal it from the world, at least till Vyāsa was older and fully able to defend himself. For once they acknowledged to the world that she was their daughter, they would have to explain why she was sent away. And that would compromise her son's safety, which neither she nor they would ever do.

Even if they recognized her, or if she told them who she was, they might send her away again in the name of safety. She might even be rebuked for risking so much by coming to see them. That thought disturbed her greatly and almost broke her spirit. She turned her mind back to the river and begged Yamunā to protect her from heartbreak.

She eagerly turned her mind to Parā-śara, imagined him on the riverbank, and felt nothing more painful than a deep, melancholy resignation that provoked a mere few minutes of tears. By now, Satya saw clearly that Parā-śara was a pure, serene sage who had long ago transcended his desire, anger, and martial spirit.

Satya-vatī felt the blood of a warrior princess flowing through her. She still needed love in her life. She loved Parā-śara, but she forbade her heart to cling to a soul so detached, so free of the romantic needs that still moved her. Still, he was the first young man of culture and stature who had noticed her, and perhaps loved her in his own distant way. He was the father of her child. But he was Parā-śara. This topic, too, must be abandoned if she was to travel happily.

Satya thought of Pearl River, the glorious royal capital she had seen through Parā-śara's powerful words. She would soon actually stand in that city. These thoughts brought her back to the celebrated birth family she had never seen. Summoning courage, she resolved that she would not let their indifference make her so. How could she not be excited to see her parents and brothers? Thus resigned to be ignored and devastated when she saw them, she journeyed on.

Her small party stopped for the night at a marina at the confluence of Yamunā and Pearl River, Śukti-matī. As they had already informed her, the chaperone couple went to bed early. Satya then steered her little boat to a remote empty dock, and paid the guard a small fee to leave it there until her return. She paid a little extra for the guard to give wrong answers if anyone asked about her. She then went to bed, rising before dawn, before her chaperones came out of their room for breakfast. She knew that breakfast was a big meal for them, and she counted on them taking considerable time at it, as they always did in Kalpi, and as they told her they would do here as well.

Before the sun rose, she boarded a ferry that went straight south to the capital. After they had traveled for over an hour, some men on the ferry began to stare at her, for she was very beautiful. To escape them, she quietly slipped off the boat at the next stop and continued south on foot toward the capital. As planned, by the time her chaperones discovered her absence, she was too far away to be overtaken.

As she walked through a particularly remote stretch of trail, two hunters suddenly emerged from the forest. Seeing her alone, they rudely blocked her way, laughing at their own vulgar jokes.

Satya-vatī's warrior blood began to boil, but the hunters mocked her sharp words and drew knives. They warned her that resistance would only cause them to do worse things. She was about to summon her Avatāra son, when the sound of a galloping horse broke the air.

"Help me!" Satya cried. Headed in another direction, the horseman quickly stopped, turned his horse, drew his sword, and dashed to her side. Seeing this finely dressed young horseman racing toward them, the hunters dropped their knives, fell to their knees, and begged him for mercy. Satya looked on in wonder. The young man was no older than her. Who was he?

"What are you doing?" he demanded of the hunters.

"Nothing at all, Your Highness," said one of the hunters. "This young lady seemed to need directions, and..."

"You are liars, rogues, and probably thieves!" Satya-vatī cried out boldly. She then turned to the young man and said, "If you are truly a prince, then forgive me for not first offering you my respects. But as you can see, the situation was a bit entangled before you most kindly intervened." Satya-vatī then bowed her head and said, "With all my heart, I thank you for your gallant rescue. I am indebted."

"Forgive you?" he said with a smile. "I am delighted to meet you. Excuse me for just a moment."

He raised his lethal sword, glared at the hunters who remained on their knees, and said, "You know my reputation. It is not false. I am very eager to send you now to the lord of death. See if he believes your story."

The prince jumped down from his horse and walked toward the men with his sword drawn. Every movement of his body evinced terrible power and consummate martial skill. The hunters begged for mercy. The prince glanced at Satya-vatī as if she was to decide the fate of those who offended her. She and the prince understood each other. With a simple nod, she asked him to spare them this time. He understood and nodded back to her. Their mutual understanding was remarkable.

The prince stood over the rogues, with his razor-sharp sword just above their heads. He said, "This kind young lady has ordered me to spare your lives. Had she so wished, you would both be dead now."

The rogues bowed to Satya-vatī, who looked away. The prince said, "Your faces are fixed in my memory. Your next offense to an innocent of this realm will be your last, I assure you. And you will not enjoy a painless death."

Terrified, the hunters bowed again, assuring the prince that there would be no other offense. He released them and they ran into the forest.

The prince, for so he was, turned back to Satya-vatī and asked, "Is there anything at all I can do for you, young lady?"

"You have probably saved my life, for which I am ever grateful. But who are you, sir? Kindly tell me to whom I owe such a debt."

"You don't know me," he said, with smiling surprise.

"I'm sorry, but I live far to the north, where sacred Yamunā flows. And you, sir, are you truly a prince?"

"I believe I am," he said, clearly fascinated with Satya-vatī. "I am Prince Matsya, son of King Vasu."

It was her brother! Her twin brother! That explained the hunter's fear. Matsya possessed a well-deserved reputation as a deadly fighter. Among the Cedi princes, he had long been her favorite for his youth and gallantry, and now she knew him to be her twin brother.

Indeed, he was as handsome as she was beautiful. As they looked more closely at each other, both were struck by their resemblance. They were twins! But only Satya knew that.

With no inkling that he even had a sister, he could not help staring at her, for their resemblance astonished him. Unwilling to leave, he gave her a friendly little bow and said, "You told me you come from the north. But who are you, young lady? And why are you traveling alone? I mean no offense. I just want to know."

By etiquette she must answer, for he had revealed his own identity to her. "I am Satya-vatī." She dreaded a question about her family.

"And your family?" he asked.

This was hard. She longed to say, "I am your long-lost sister. We are twins! I often thought of you, even before I knew you to be my dear brother."

But she had sworn not to reveal her true identity, lest she cause trouble to her family and her son. To her mortification, all she could say was, "I was raised in a village." And in barely audible tones, she added, "I was raised by the head of a fishing village, and his wife."

"Raised by them?" the prince said, intrigued. "So they are not your natural parents?"

"I have reason to believe they are not," Satya-vatī said, seeing that her brother shared her sharp intelligence, and that now, to her shame, he must think her to be an illegitimate child. This was getting worse.

But Prince Matsya seemed not to notice. Rather, he said, "You do speak very well, far more like a brāhmaṇī than a fishing girl."

"I studied with learned sages near my village."

"Remarkable!" he said. "I've never heard of such a case. He kept looking at her, for there was indeed a striking resemblance between them, one that only she understood. He apologized for staring, and said, "In addition to our startling resemblance, which I trust you too have noticed, I see that you have a…well, a sort of aura about you, as if you were glowing. I am most anxious to know more about you. I would be grateful if you would kindly tell me where you are going?"

"To the great capital, Pearl River," she replied.

"Yes, the great capital. Have you been there before?"

"No, never, but I've heard much about it."

"Yes, of course," he said. "Satya-vatī, you really must forgive me for staring, we do have a most uncanny resemblance."

"Indeed we do. And you need not apologize."

"Well, you are most welcome to hop on my horse and come with me to the capital."

"I would gladly do so, I assure you," she said. "But you know how people would talk."

"I will simply tell everyone that I rescued you from rogues."

"Yes, but people might not believe it. I truly believe you to be a prince of excellent character, but you know that common people love to gossip about royalty."

"Indeed they do," he said. "Excellent observation. You are right. People certainly would talk. I admire your caution. But I cannot leave you in this way. You must take my horse. I'll find another one on the road."

Satya-vatī smiled and almost laughed at this proposal. He smiled with her. They were friends.

"Thank you," she said, "but I've never ridden a horse in my life, and I don't think you have time to teach me now."

He smiled again. "You are not an ordinary girl," he said.

She sighed, longing to say, "I am your own sister. I have long admired you. We have every right to travel together."

"But why do you travel alone," he insisted, "and how will you get to the city? Forgive my intrusion, but I am sincerely concerned about you. Indeed, you are a citizen of the realm, and therefore by Dharma, I am responsible to see that you reach your destination safely."

"Thank you so much, Prince Matsya. You are a most worthy prince of the realm." Then without technically lying, she said, "The couple accompanying me lost the trail and we were separated."

This was true because they did indeed lose her trail. "Anyway," she said with determination, "I'm sure Viṣṇu will protect me, as he did now by sending you."

"I suppose he will," Matsya said, clearly pleased with her spirit and intrigued by her faith in Viṣṇu. "And I hope," he added, "that I am pleasing Viṣṇu by helping you. Indeed, I really must help you reach the capital. I can't just leave you alone like this. But tell me, where will you stay in the capital?"

"I confess I didn't think of that," she admitted.

"Let me guess," he said, "Viṣṇu will provide you a place, right?"

"Yes," she said. They both laughed. They heard the jangle and thud of an oxcart heading their way. The prince walked to the cart. A man and woman sat in front. They stopped at the sight of the prince and bowed. Satya-vatī watched as the prince conversed with them. They all nodded and smiled and Matsya walked back to her.

"It is all settled," he said. "This kind couple will take you to Pearl River. I offered to pay for your food and lodging on the way but they insisted with insurmountable good will that they would be happy to provide for you. They are good people. You will be safe with them. When you get to the capital, come to the palace and ask for me. You must promise to do that."

She smiled and promised. He pulled from his finger a gold ring with his name engraved on it. "Show this at the palace gates and you will be admitted," he said. "I will reach there, God willing, long before you and I will inform the gatekeepers."

As he accompanied her to the oxcart, he said, "Remember, you promised to come and see me. Viṣṇu won't like it if you don't keep your promise!"

She laughed and renewed her promise. He laughed with genuine good will and said, "There is something special about you. Anyway, you said you were indebted to me, and you will pay your debt by visiting me."

So earnestly, yet so teasingly did he claim his debt that Satya had to smile and promise yet again to visit him. It was settled. They bowed cordially to each other.

He mounted his fine horse, they exchanged friendly waves, and he rode swiftly away. Satya-vatī watched in wonder till he vanished over the horizon. This sudden meeting with her twin, Matsya, thrilled her. Surely Viṣṇu had arranged such an improbable meeting. Yet the need to hide her identity from those with whom she ought to be most open and intimate frustrated and saddened her.

She climbed into the oxcart with the help of its owners. Sincere introductions were made on both sides, and she was on her way to Pearl River.

She thought repeatedly of her encounter with Matsya. By contact with the Avatāra, she had been transformed. But only the godly could see it. Matsya had seen it. He even said she glowed. As the slow cart moved toward the capital, she anxiously anticipated her next meeting with her brother, indeed, with her loving parents, and all her family.

CHAPTER 14

On the road to Pearl River, Satya-vatī heard from villagers along the way that all five Cedi princes — her brothers — had come to the capital to meet with their father — her father. And her mother!

But all her emotion was pathetic and useless. Even if she revealed herself to her parents, they could not publicly welcome her as their daughter, for then they would have to explain why she was sent away at birth. That might put the Avatāra child and herself in danger. Her situation was hopeless. Satya would not stay long in the capital. She could not bear many days of this anxiety.

What if she revealed herself to her parents and her visit angered or disturbed them? They might consider her irresponsible, foolhardy, or even deny her as their daughter. That she could not endure.

Despite all these horrid scenarios that assaulted her mind, Satya-vatī did hold in her heart a rational hope for a more positive outcome. If nothing else, she would see the fabled city. She would see all her family. After all, she would always cherish her brief meeting with Matsya, despite the confusion and concealment. She could never wish that their brief meeting had not happened. That settled it. She must see Pearl River and her family.

As she neared the city, the road widened into an elegant avenue, shaded on both sides by flowering trees. Here she insisted on getting down from the oxcart. The kind couple insisted that they arrange a place for her. She insisted it was not necessary.

She thanked them profusely and got down. She needed time alone, and she was sure that she would find a place to stay among all these kind people. She carried her few possessions in a cloth bag. Ladies and gentlemen in horse-drawn carriages passed her as she walked on a pedestrian lane covered with handsome paving stones.

She had seen the city once before through Parā-śara's words. She joyfully recognized the white marble spires that rose above the trees; music and fragrance were in the air. Green parks beckoned her; lovely houses charmed her. Laughing children played, opulent markets bustled, fountains cooled the air, and everywhere she saw joyful people in fine clothes and jewels greeting one another, living in peace and plenty. Satya sighed. It all lifted her spirits. This was truly Pearl River, the grand capital of Cedi. She fixed her mind in Viṣṇu and did not even worry about her simple country dress. There must be a greater plan.

She walked along the very river where her father rescued her mother! She saw the remains of Mount Kolāhala! And there on the riverbank her parents first gazed into each other's eyes and fell in love.

The towering Royal Palace came into view. Built of finely carved red sandstone, and marble of various colors, it shone in the light of a tropical sun. But now, the full gravity of where she was, and what she was about to do, struck her and her courage failed. She resolved not to enter the palace. If by Viṣṇu's will the royal family came out, or passed her way, she would see them. She would make no endeavor. Fear of rejection, of humiliation, paralyzed her. She sat and worried.

But then, loud trumpets blown by soldiers atop the palace walls shattered her brooding meditation. A deep voice cried out, "Their Majesties open their doors to the people of Cedi! All who seek their audience with petitions or gifts may enter now."

The palace gates swung open, and orderly citizens, politely greeting one another, entered the gates into the palace courtyard. She had only to join their number. In a few moments, she would be facing her birth parents, the most celebrated couple in the world. She could not move. Too much could go wrong, and what could really go right? No, she would not go in. She couldn't. If she was meant to enter, then Viṣṇu would send her a sign. She looked up to heaven. Yes, let Viṣṇu send her a sign.

"This must be Viṣṇu!" cried a voice. Startled, Satya looked around and saw Prince Matsya approaching her. His quick, confident strides brought him there in a moment. "I was hoping to see you here," he said with enthusiasm so artless that she could not doubt his sincerity. "How long have you been here?"

"I arrived but an hour ago."

"I see. And where are you staying?"

"I don't really know. I didn't think about it," she stammered.

Well, Satya thought with self-reproach, my clumsy reply and lack of a plan certainly go well with my coarse country clothes. What will he think of me?

"Really?" he said. "Alone in the city with no place to stay. Well, we will fix that. But for now, come with me into the palace."

"Oh, but I—"

"Don't be shy. My parents like to personally welcome visitors. Let's surprise them, since you are practically my twin." He laughed at the idea. Satya didn't know whether she would laugh or cry. But she could not refuse him. She could not deny that Viṣṇu had sent the sign she had promised to follow.

With her heart beating too quickly, and not feeling the ground beneath her feet, she walked side by side with Prince Matsya into the palace. The guards and heralds bowed their heads to him and stared at her. She knew why they were staring. She didn't belong here.

"You are making quite an impression," Prince Matsya whispered to her. "People are impressed by your beauty and grace."

She shook her head but did not speak. And all at once she was inside the palace. A line of citizens waited patiently to speak with their rulers. A wide space separated those waiting from those actually speaking to the royal couple. Satya-vatī saw that this arrangement kept each conversation with the rulers strictly private.

She instinctively headed for the back of the line. Prince Matsya laughed at her and said, "We're not going to wait in line, Satya-vatī. I have a seat up front."

"Oh no," she said, "I cannot approach your parents."

"But why? You look like me. They'll like you for that, if nothing else," he said with a laugh. Satya considered running for the door but concluded that such a move would be absurd. As these thoughts swirled in her mind, Prince Matsya had not stopped leading her forward, and she suddenly found herself standing in front of King Vasu and Queen Girikā. She looked down at her feet.

"Prince Matsya," said the queen, "who is this guest that you've brought to us?" The sound of the queen's voice shook Satya's heart. It was the same voice of the young Girikā that fell in love with Vasu.

The prince briefly explained how he met Satya-vatī and saved her from two criminals.

"Oh, you mentioned that, and now the girl has come to our city. Please, dear girl, lift your head. You needn't be afraid here. My son told me that you are a beautiful young lady."

"Indeed, she is," Prince Matsya said, "although she has suddenly become so shy that you can't even see her face. But I saved a surprise for you both."

"A surprise?" the king said. "And what would that be?"

"Simply this, that by a most improbable coincidence, this lovely girl looks like my twin."

A complete silence followed these words. Matsya apparently didn't notice. He nudged her and whispered in her ear, "Satya-vatī, look up! Let them see you!"

She had no choice. With heart stopped, barely breathing, she lifted her eyes toward her parents.

Her resemblance to Matsya was too striking to be misunderstood by her parents. The king stared and clenched the arms of his throne as if to hold himself steady.

"Oh my God!" cried the queen, trembling on her throne. Matsya looked on in confusion.

Struggling for composure, King Vasu said, "Forgive our surprise, young lady, but...you do...look like our son's twin. Kindly tell us who you are? Where is your home? Who is your family? Please tell us, if you will."

Facing her parents, feeling herself to be in a dream, Satya decided to reveal herself in words that only her parents could understand.

"Your Majesties," she said, bowing to them with folded hands, "a Vedic sage once told me that although I grew up in a humble fishing village, he saw me as a princess...though perhaps a neglected one."

Stunned, her parents stared but could not speak. Prince Matsya, seeing that something very serious was taking place, became grave. His eyes darted from one parent to another and back to Satya.

Overwhelmed with emotion, Satya burst into tears. Queen Girikā was about to rush off her throne to comfort her, but King Vasu gently held her arm, and made a quick sign that only the queen and her daughter noticed. Girikā sat back on her throne, fighting back her own tears.

King Vasu, feigning calm in a way that perhaps only Satya-vatī could detect, then said to Prince Matsya, "Please escort this young lady to the palace gardens, and see that she is comfortable in every way. I cannot neglect the citizens who have come to see me, but as soon as we are done here, your mother and I will speak with this girl in our private quarters. Is that clear?"

"Yes sir, very clear." Matsya said, astonished by his father's words. No one but close family had admittance to the private quarters of the king and queen.

Matsya gently took Satya-vatī's arm and led her out of the throne room, through splendid halls, to the most beautiful gardens she had ever seen. As they sat together by a lotus pond, he offered to bring refreshments, but she declined. He then looked at her seriously and said, "Satya, what happened in there? What is going on?"

What could she say?

"Satya!" he said, "You weren't this disturbed on the highway when those killers attacked you. What is happening here?"

Satya-vatī took a deep breath, looked into her brother's eyes, and said softly, "There is something. And with all my heart I want to tell you. Believe me I do. But I can only tell you with the permission of your parents."

Moved and amazed by her words, he said gently, "You know my parents?"

"Yes, I mean, no. I think they want to speak to me…"

"They certainly do. They almost fell off their thrones when they saw you. Satya-vatī, who are you?"

She blushed and said, "Please, when I see them, I will ask if I am free to tell you. Oh, Matsya, I mean Prince Matsya…"

"No, please, just Matsya."

"Thank you. Matsya, you have been so kind to me. You are a prince and I am…" She hesitated.

"Yes, who you are seems to be the question. But I will not ask you this again until my parents authorize you to tell me. Agreed?"

Satya-vatī breathed an audible sigh of relief. "Yes, that's perfect. Thank you. Can I ask you about something else?"

Matsya nodded graciously. "Yes, of course. It's just so remarkable how strongly I feel I know you. And obviously, you are my twin." He said this playfully, without any notion that he was speaking a literal truth. Satya smiled and asked, "Where are your brothers? I've heard from the citizens that all five of you are here in the capital."

"Yes, we're all here. The other four went out riding. They should be back before dark. We've all come together because our father is going to formally assign kingdoms to those sons who do not yet have them. It seems that I am to receive a very special assignment. Are you interested?"

"Yes!" Satya-vatī exclaimed. "Most interested! Tell me, please, if you can."

Encouraged by her response, Matsya said, "I am in the process of founding a new kingdom."

"A new kingdom? Please, tell me about it."

"Gladly. I know I can trust you. I am building a new capital in a somewhat distant region northwest of here. It is roughly a fifteen-day march from Pearl River, the border of the great western desert."

Satya playfully asked the prince if she could guess the location of his new capital. Fascinated, he eagerly agreed. She quickly gathered twigs and thin branches from nearby trees, kneeled on the manicured lawn, and constructed a simple map, as she learned to do on the sand of the brāhmaṇa village in Kalpi.

Matsya watched in amazement. Satya then stated precisely where his capital would be.

Matsya shook his head in wonder. "How did you do that?"

"Simple geometry. Do you have a name for your new kingdom?"

"Now that is a bit embarrassing." He laughed. "My father is so pleased that I am willing to start a new kingdom, and forego for now the convenience and comfort of an established realm, that he insists on naming the kingdom after me — the Kingdom of Matsya. I hope you don't think it was my idea, and that I am hopelessly vain."

Satya-vatī laughed and assured him that she would never think any such thing about him. He was pleased and laughed with her. She was about to compliment the royal family on their lovely gardens, when Matsya signaled her to turn around, and said, "Someone is entering the garden."

Satya-vatī turned. A young prince about twelve years old, tall and strong for his age, stood at the garden entrance. Meeting Satya's eyes, he offered a curt bow and said, "Uncle Matsya, may I join you?"

"Hey, Trīya! Yes, of course. Come join us."

"I don't want to bother you," the youth said, looking intently at Satya-vatī.

Matsya waved away his scruples. "Don't be silly, come and join us."

The boy approached and gave another curt bow to Satya-vatī."

"You are such a gentleman," she said. "It's a pleasure to meet you, Prince Trīya."

The boy smiled and again looked carefully at Satya. She felt he was studying her.

Matsya turned to Satya and said, "This boy's father is my oldest brother, Bṛhad-ratha."

Satya-vatī's heart trembled. Did Bṛhad-ratha have a second son? Anxious to find out, she said, "The boy has an unusual name, Trīya. I don't think I've heard it before."

"Oh, that's just a nickname," Matsya said. "It's short for Bhrātrīya."

"Of course, Bhrātrīya, nephew," Satya said, struggling to conceal her anxiety.

"Exactly," the boy said boldly. "My real name is Jarā-sandha. I am the first son and heir of King Bṛhad-ratha. I am proud to be the third generation of our dynasty."

These words were clearly directed to her. Satya-vatī struggled to remain composed. Any sign of confusion or weakness would reveal her knowledge, possibly endangering herself and her family. She remembered Viṣṇu and felt strength within. Steadying herself, she said with a passable semblance of composure, "Jarā-sandha, I am delighted to meet you."

He looked at her plain dress and smiled with proud condescension, as if looking upon a low-level servant.

"What is your name?" he asked, staring into her eyes, searching for clues to the reason for her presence there.

"I am Satya-vatī," she said. "I am a simple girl from North Cedi. Your uncle, Prince Matsya, rescued me from highway robbers, and kindly invited me to the palace."

She saw that he did not consider her explanation to be the whole story. He continued to study her. Feeling most uncomfortable under his probing gaze, she decided to change the subject and said, "It is a real honor to be the third generation of such a noble family. I am very happy for you."

"Thank you," he said, still suspicious.

Matsya then began to chat with his nephew about ordinary family affairs. Jarā-sandha held up his part of the conversation, but he kept glancing at her. With alarm, she realized that even as he chatted with his uncle, Jarā-sandha sought to enter her mind and discover her secrets. Keeping a calm exterior, but alarmed at his mental power, Satya-vatī silently appealed to Viṣṇu, and felt his strength protecting her mind. Jarā-sandha could not penetrate her thoughts. She detected disappointment in his eyes. She smiled at him, and he smiled back as if to say, "I will defeat you. You will not escape."

Matsya said, "One day Jarā-sandha will inherit a mighty kingdom from his father. One day, he will rule Magadha."

"I congratulate your nephew," she said. "That is a great honor. I'm sure he will rule wisely."

"I'm sure he will," Matsya said. Jarā-sandha smiled and thanked his uncle, without looking at Satya-vatī.

A royal herald entered the garden and informed Prince Matsya that his parents would now receive Satya-vatī. Matsya was to personally bring her. They would follow the herald to the meeting place.

"I will also go," Jarā-sandha said.

"Forgive me, Your Highness," the herald said, "but I received strict orders that only Prince Matsya and Satya-vatī are to come."

Jarā-sandha suppressed his anger, smiled, and nodded. He said to his uncle, "With your permission, Uncle, I will go to military practice." Then with a glance at Satya-vatī, he said, "A warrior must be invincible against all foes, even the Devas."

CHAPTER 15

To Satya's and Matsya's surprise, the herald led them not to the royal couple's quarters, but toward a huge lawn behind the palace.

"Oh, you're in luck," Prince Matsya said merrily. "There's been a change of plans. It seems we're going for a ride in the crystal aircraft! My parents must really like you."

Indeed, as they approached the lawn and passed a palace wall that had obstructed their view, Satya saw the aircraft. She gasped in wonder, for it resembled a small palace and hovered just above rich, green grass. Thrilled, Satya-vatī went eagerly forward with her twin brother, who, she knew, felt an increasingly strong connection to her, though he did not know why.

The king and queen and their other four sons now emerged from the palace and strode boldly toward the aircraft. Satya easily recognized Bṛhad-ratha, the eldest and most imposing of the sons. As he came near, he called out and waved to Matsya, who waved back and added a humorous remark.

Satya-vatī studied the five princes with admiration. Vasu's sons were all energetic. They were wise warrior kings who built a dynasty with their father. Indra had promised Vasu an imperial dynasty, and now she saw its leaders before her eyes. She bowed her head to Indra, for the Deva king had empowered her family.

Just as when Parā-śara first showed her the aircraft, a crystal plank came down. The king motioned for all to board. Satya-vatī could hardly believe where she was and what was about to happen. As she walked into the main room of the aircraft, the furnishings dazzled her. Yet it was all done in good taste and without ostentation. All around the craft she saw weapons so advanced that ordinary people would call them mystical.

Within her heart, she called out to dear goddess Yamunā, begging to be protected from saying foolish words, or doing anything that would make her family think ill of her. If we fly high enough, Satya thought, I may see you, dear Yamunā.

She thought of her foster parents and prayed for their well-being. How could she ever explain to them where she was right now? They would hardly believe her. She thought of Parā-śara and his solemn promise that good fortune would come to her.

Satya could not resist walking about the perimeter of the large room, looking through the floor-to-ceiling crystal windows. Even more than when she first saw it, she admired the capital skyline, with its fine turrets and towers, and the flowering forests that surrounded the city.

Matsya whispered to her, "My parents want to see you in their private chamber. It's that way."

"Oh no," she said, suddenly nervous. "Come with me, Matsya. I can't see them alone."

"You have nothing to fear," he said, still whispering. "They were quite emphatic that you come alone. I long to know what is going on with you and my parents. But I'll wait. You can't make them call you twice. Etiquette!"

"Of course," she said, hurrying with a waiting herald to the private chamber of King Vasu and Queen Girikā. Her heart pounded and she stopped breathing. She was going alone to face her parents. All her careful plans for this moment fled her mind. She did not feel the floor beneath her. She entered and immediately bowed.

The king and queen sat on seats worthy of their position. Queen Girikā gave an anxious smile, and motioned for her to sit on a seat facing the royal couple, who seemed as nervous as Satya-vatī.

She bowed again, thanked them, and quickly took her seat. What would they say?

"Dear girl," said the queen in a gentle voice, "when we first met in the palace, you told us that a Vedic sage spoke to you about your true identity. Did I hear you correctly?"

"Yes, Your Majesty," Satya said, trying hard not to tremble.

"Did that sage forbid you to tell me and the king all that he told you? If he did, I will respect his wish, though I hope he did not tell you that."

"Your Majesty, the sage did not forbid me to tell you all he told me. I want to tell you everything. I want that very much."

Tears now streamed from Satya's eyes. She apologized and tried to wipe her eyes in a dignified way, but her hands could hardly find her eyes. The queen said, "My dear girl, you have done nothing wrong."

The king looked at his wife, then at Satya, and back to his wife. He seemed anxious that his wife do the talking. When Satya had calmed herself, the queen said, "Dear Satya-vatī, the sage who spoke to you — was it Parā-śara?"

"Yes, it was."

"And what did he tell you about your identity?"

"He told me that I am your daughter, and the king is my father. You sent me away at birth, to protect me from Asuras, because I had been chosen to bring an Avatāra into this world."

Queen Girikā seemed about to rush to Satya, but her husband held up his hand, and whispered into her ear. She sat back in her seat.

"Forgive us," the king said, "but the Asuras may be anywhere, and some of them are even powerful yogīs who possess a power called kāma-rūpa, by which they can take on any form they wish. It is therefore my sacred duty to humanity, to the Devas, and not least of all to my own daughter, to ask you a question."

"Of course," Satya-vatī said. "Please."

"The question is simple. Can you tell me something that only my daughter and Parā-śara could possibly know? Perhaps a secret that my daughter shared with the sage, or that he discovered in her mind."

"Oh, that's easy," Satya-vatī said with a sigh of relief. "I know just what you are hinting at. Parā-śara knew my most precious secret, one that I never revealed to anyone."

"And what is that?" The queen leaned forward anxiously.

"It is this. From time to time, and always on my birthday, you and the king flew over my village in this very crystal aircraft. I thought it was a guardian star. But it was you, my parents, coming to see me and to watch over me. When Parā-śara told me my most precious secret, something I told no one, then I knew that he was truly a great sage and I could trust him fully. And I knew that you, my parents, truly loved me."

Queen Girikā now rushed to Satya-vatī and held her in her arms as if she would never let go. The mother's tears bathed the head of her child. "You are my daughter!" she cried, caressing Satya's head with her hands. "You are my only daughter. I knew it as soon as I saw you, but I could not speak until you confirmed it. These are the times we live in, but you understand all that. Oh, how I missed you all these years! I thought my heart would break."

Satya-vatī wept in her arms. Holding her daughter tight, Girikā said, "My only daughter. My only daughter. How I missed you! Now go to your father."

Vasu stood waiting for her with open arms. Satya-vatī rushed to him and as he embraced her, he said, "My dear child, if we acted wrongly, if we caused you unnecessary pain and suffering, we beg you to forgive us. We feared for your life and we loved you too much to risk any harm to you. Ultimately, we acted on the order of Indra himself. Your mother and I flew over your village many times just to see you. Our hearts were breaking, but we had to follow Indra, who knows more than we do. How could we defy him, knowing that we might be putting you in great danger? We could never have forgiven ourselves. But can you forgive us?"

These words from her parents deeply moved Satya-vatī. Holding her father tight, she said through her tears that she did not blame them for anything.

Girikā said, "We must ascend now or the palace staff will think it strange that we are still here and they will come to check on us. Let us get away, where we can be a family in peace."

"Yes," the king said, "we'll go now. But first, Satya-vatī, is there anything that you wish to ask us?"

Satya thought, and said, "Perhaps only this; how did you know that the Asura beasts were going to attack the brāhmaṇas in Kalpi? How did you come so quickly?"

"First, I always monitor your area, because of my special concern for you. Also, Indra gave me the power to hear the cries of brāhmaṇas from afar. And in this case, he warned me of a possible attack in your area. And of course, he knew the importance of bringing the Avatāra safely to this world."

Satya-vatī smiled. "But now," her father said, "we must leave, as your mother said. Dear girl, when we stop in a secluded place, we will explain everything to your brothers." He then opened the door for the ladies and accompanied them into the main hall. His sons stared at them, for all three were in an emotional state.

Before his sons could say a word, the king said, "Let us depart." Everyone took a seat and at Girikā's behest, Satya-vatī sat beside her. Vasu focused intensely and the aircraft rose silently into the air. Despite its speed, Satya felt no discomfort; indeed, she felt no motion. She saw below the entire city, with its surrounding fields and forests.

"Satya-vatī has never seen the capital from the air," the king said. "We will stop here for a moment."

Satya gasped in wonder as she looked down on the splendid city, with its bright, wide ribbon of river threading its way around palaces and parks. "Is there any place in the world like this?" she asked.

"Oh, there is a greater city," Vasu replied, "the imperial Kuru capital, Hastinā-pura. Now, our Cedi dynasty dominates the world. But for centuries the Kurus stood above all other kingdoms. Their imperial city, Hastinā-pura, is legendary."

"Of course I've heard of it," Satya said. "People say it's like the Deva realm on Earth."

"I went there once," Matsya said, "and all that you heard is true."

"Oh, if just once in my life, I could see Hastinā-pura!" Satya said, and her family smiled at the innocent enthusiasm of a country girl.

"Perhaps one day," Girikā said, "we can introduce you to King Śan-tanu. We are his distant cousins, and he will be eager to make our acquaintance. I'm sure of that."

Satya-vatī bowed and thanked her.

"Where are we going, Father?" Bṛhad-ratha asked.

"Where would you like to go?" Vasu asked Satya-vatī.

"I can't imagine," she said. She thought of asking to see the great Himālaya mountains where her son was living, but thought it best not to mention Dvaipāyana. She thought of the celebrated Kuru capital of Hastinā-pura, but her family might feel a rivalry with that ancient dynasty. She thought of her own village with her foster parents. But having just met her real parents, it might seem indelicate of her to ask to go there. So she turned to Bṛhad-ratha and said, "Perhaps you can suggest a destination."

"We have serious topics to discuss. So let us fly to the Southern Sea, where Lord Rāma built his mystic bridge. Rāma will inspire and guide us."

"So be it," the king said. "We will be there shortly. I will land on the beach." The aircraft turned and headed straight for the Vindhya hills that divide North and South. Satya-vatī went to a large window and stared in wonder at forests, farms, and rivers that rushed by below.

As they crossed the Narmadā River and the Vindhya peaks, the subcontinent narrowed. She saw the great seas that border Bharata to the East and West. Strikingly faceted green hills rose on each coast.

As they flew toward the southern tip of the subcontinent, Satya had a few pleasant minutes to speak alone with Matsya. They talked and joked like old friends, as her parents looked on approvingly.

Then, sooner than she thought possible, the crystal aircraft floated down onto a wide and deserted island beach near the southern tip of the subcontinent. This was the region of Rameśvara. The five princes eagerly disembarked and at the queen's urging, Matsya and three of his brothers ran to sport in the sea. Only the eldest son, Bṛhad-ratha, looked grave. He walked pensively behind them. Satya-vatī surmised that only the king and queen and their eldest son knew the identity of Jarā-sandha and the danger he posed. The others must believe that the royal family had stopped the Asuras, that now was a time for peaceful living and casual governance.

Satya-vatī stayed behind at the earnest request of her parents. As they sat alone in the crystal aircraft, Satya's mother grasped her hands and said, "My dear girl, forgive me, but I must inquire about a most delicate but crucial matter."

Satya encouraged the queen to speak anything that concerned her. The queen nodded, glanced at the king, and then said to her daughter, "Tell me, my dearest girl, is the Avatāra born? Does he live safely on this planet?"

Even before she spoke her reply, Satya-vatī's spontaneous, heartfelt smile told the good news. Each parent grasped one of her hands, as she said, "The Avatāra has come indeed and he is safe! Parā-śara has personally taken him to a most secluded, concealed āśrama. There the child quickly gathers his powers and will soon be invulnerable to any Asura attack. He is safe!"

The emperor and empress gave out a cry of joy and embraced their daughter. How grateful and glad Satya was then, for doing her duty despite her personal struggle.

Now the five princes shouted insistently for their parents and Satyavatī to come down to the beach. The king waved to them, and in a few moments, the entire family was united in that sacred place. The royal couple and their daughter sat on the beach and watched the mighty princes sport in the water. All five were big, strong, and handsome, and they clearly enjoyed one another's company. Satya saw that it was a loving family, and this thought pained her as she realized what she had lost for so many years. But now was not the time to lament and she banished all sad ideas from her mind.

Balmy breezes skimmed the glassy blue waters, bringing the scent and flavor of the sea, and ruffling her hair. Tall coconut trees swayed to and fro.

As she sat on soft sand with her loving parents, in the midst of tropical splendor, Satya did not lament. She focused on present great fortune. She was with her family! Her parents hinted they would reveal her identity to her brothers. She would gain five loving brothers. This thought filled her heart with so much joy that she now had to contend with giddy bliss, not lamentation.

Finally, Vasu called his sons. They came running and shouting. Only Bṛhad-ratha was silent. Their wet bodies dried quickly in the southern heat. They changed clothes in a coconut grove, and sat around their parents, who kept Satya next to them.

"As you know," the king began, "most serious matters require our attention. You know why I summoned you. The time has come for the four younger sons to be crowned as kings in their respective realms, like their eldest brother, Bṛhad-ratha. And as I always said, the five sons together will rule Cedi when your mother and I are gone."

The sons nodded, but Satya saw that her presence at an intimate family discussion puzzled them. Vasu said, "Before I begin those topics of ascension, I will mention another issue of grave importance. Naturally, you are wondering why this beautiful young lady, Satya-vatī, sits with us as if she were part of our family. You may wonder why your mother and I give her such special attention."

"I confess," Bṛhad-ratha said, "that her presence here amazes me, considering the gravity and intimacy of this family discussion. You know we mean no offense to you, nor to the young lady. But we are exceedingly astonished by her presence here."

"You have every reason to be astonished," the king said. "I take no offense, and I believe the young lady takes none either." He looked at Satya, who said, "Of course I take no offense, Your Majesty. I know why I am here, and I am astonished myself. But forgive me if I say too much."

"Not at all," the king replied, pleased with her self-confidence. "But perhaps your mother had better explain." He looked at Girikā and asked, "Is that all right with you?"

The queen nodded. "Dear boys, surely you noticed that Satya-vatī bears a striking resemblance to Matsya, as if she were his twin."

The brothers all said they had indeed noticed.

"The reason is simple," the queen said, as tears streamed down her cheeks. As her five sons stared in anxious anticipation, Girikā said, "Dear sons, Satya-vatī so resembles Matsya because she is Matsya's twin sister."

The brothers gazed at their sister in utter astonishment.

"To save your sister's life," the queen said, "and the life of an Avatāra destined to be her son, your father and I were forced to send her away. Because of the importance of her mission, she was in grave danger."

After swearing the boys to secrecy, which she knew they would keep on their lives, Girikā explained how Indra and Śacī visited the king and queen and explained that Satya-vatī had been chosen to bring to this world an Avatāra who would play a key role in defeating the Asuras. To prevent this from happening, the Asuras would stop at nothing. Because of the importance of this Avatāra in the fight to save Earth, this girl would be in greater danger than the Cedi princes. Thus, to protect Satya-vatī, she must be sent to a remote place that Asuras could not suspect. Girikā praised Satya's foster parents, about whom she had heard from Parā-śara, but emphasized how much the girl had suffered despite their love. Girikā narrated in graphic detail the travails of her daughter. Vasu and his sons wept with compassion.

The queen then revealed that Satya-vatī and a great sage, chosen by the Devas and by Viṣṇu himself, successfully brought the Avatāra into this world.

The king turned to his daughter and said, "I cannot express how proud we are of you. You did a great service for the world. You sacrificed so much. I'm sure that your family is anxious to do all we can to make it up to you."

The five brothers applauded and loudly confirmed their father's words. "You are a true heroine, Satya-vatī," Bṛhad-ratha said. "You have done more than your brothers to save this planet."

Matsya could not contain himself. Rushing up to his twin sister, he embraced her, lifted her off her feet with his strong arms, and whirled her around, shouting, "I knew it! I knew it was something like this!"

A glance from his father reminded him that the family had grave topics to discuss. Matsya put Satya down, apologized with a smile, and took his seat. But before the meeting could proceed, even before Satya could take her seat, the other four brothers embraced her and pledged their love and service. The queen wept to see this. Satya-vatī was happy beyond what she had ever imagined possible.

There followed much conversation, in which everyone competed for her attention, to tell her from their heart how much they regretted her past travails, and how ecstatic they were to have her back with the family. Everyone wanted to know everything about her. Everyone felt they already knew her.

Their attention turned to Satya's Avatāra son. Here, their curiosity, heightened by hope that this Avatāra heralded a most auspicious and victorious future, led to many earnest pleas for information. Satya told all she knew, conscientiously giving attention to each member of the family. Finally, in reply to their insistent invitations, she expressed her joyful hope to visit all their kingdoms as soon as was practical.

Satya-vatī felt as if she had never been separated from her family. Yet she preserved in her heart a place for love and gratitude toward the stepparents who raised her from infancy.

At last, Vasu called the family to order, declaring that they would now discuss grave issues. They all sat around the king. "It is fitting," he began, "now that our family is reunited in this sacred place, that we face together the greatest challenge of our lives."

These were serious words indeed for a royal family that had known only triumph and glory. King Vasu continued, "It is fitting to discuss our greatest challenge here because in this region, the greatest king, Lord Rāma, vanquished most powerful Asuras, like Rāvaṇa. Let us first seek Rāma's blessings."

All bowed their heads to King Rāma, the divine monarch. King Vasu then continued. "I have secured for my five sons five kingdoms. We have agreed that each son will rule his own realm, and all five will govern Cedi when I am gone. Indra himself approves this plan. Our dream has always been to unite the world in peace and prosperity. However, we now have a serious problem. And for that reason, an Avatāra has come."

The king paused. Not a sound was heard. He looked at his queen, at each of his sons, and at Satya-vatī.

Vasu continued, "As you know, Lord Indra empowered our family, with its base in Cedi, to neutralize the Asura invasion. For some time, we have succeeded. But Indra warned me that the Asuras are patient, and are gathering strength."

All eyes fixed on the king. He took a deep breath, glanced at his eldest son, Bṛhad-ratha, and said, "Long ago, Indra warned me that Asuras would take birth in leading kingdoms, in an attempt to inherit the Earth. I expected this. However, I confess to you all that I did not suspect the mightiest Asura of all to boldly take birth in our family, and inherit its power. Yet that is now happening. When Indra told me this awful news, I shared it only with the queen. I also told my eldest son, Bṛhad-ratha, because the Asura leader, Vipra-citti, has taken birth in our family as Bṛhad-ratha's son and heir, Jarā-sandha. The Asuras will inherit a leading role in the very empire created by Indra to stop the Asura invasion."

Queen Girikā wept. Bṛhad-ratha hung his head in shame, as if he blamed himself for the Asura's birth in his family. The four younger princes gaped in disbelief. Satya-vatī silently implored Viṣṇu to save her family, and the Earth, from the looming disaster.

"Oh Lord!" cried Kuśāmba. "My kingdom, Kauśāmbī, borders that of Bṛhad-ratha. When we are gone, Asuras will probably attack my family first! What can we do?"

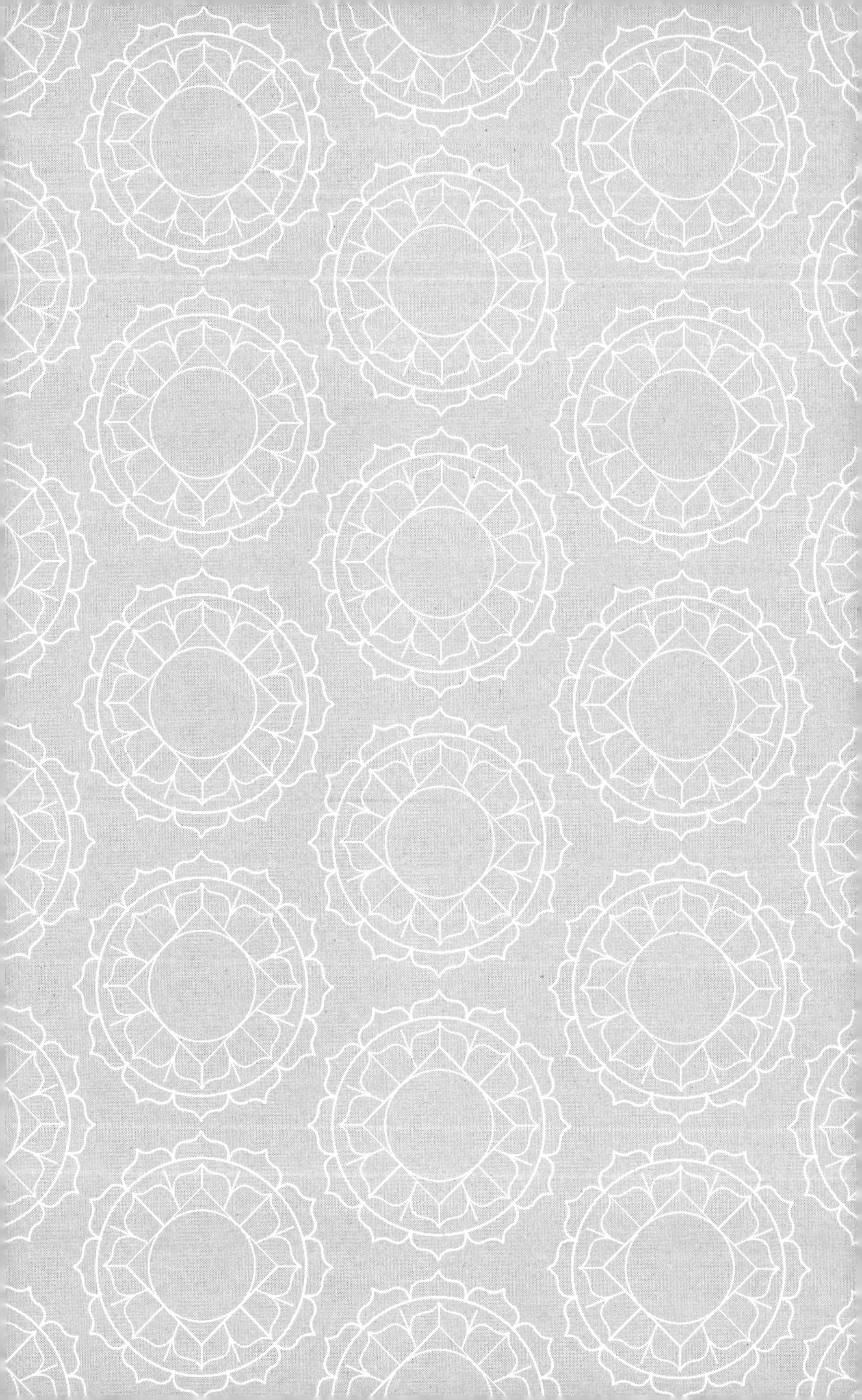

CHAPTER 16

As the general mood turned from joy to horror, King Vasu said to his second son, Kuśāmba, "Please calm down. For now, we are safe; our dynasty is strong. We have time to make a plan. Jarā-sandha knows that by Dharma, he will inherit the kingdom of Magadha. He is proud of our dynasty and does not want to weaken it. He need only act like a good son and grandson, and the kingdom is his. He will not give us any legal reason to deny him his inheritance. Once he takes power, he will act more freely, and that is the greatest threat to the world. But an Avatāra has come, and I'm sure that Viṣṇu himself will come if the world is truly in danger."

"But why didn't you tell us sooner?" Matsya said to King Vasu. "You should have told us."

"It is my fault," Bṛhad-ratha said. "I urged our father not to tell my brothers, because I foolishly thought I could change my son. As you know, I had failed to produce an heir, and this threatened our young dynasty. I was depressed. I even thought of renouncing my position as eldest son. But then a brāhmaṇa blessed me to have a son. Now I fear that the brāhmaṇa was himself an agent of the Asuras. Anyway, Indra informed our father who my son was, and of course Father told me. We knew that Indra himself failed to kill the Asura when he was still an embryo. So what could we do? He was an affectionate child, and I felt we had to *try* to change him before we turned all the family against him. As he grew, we saw that nothing we could do would change him. By that time, I feared that if Jarā-sandha knew that the family opposed him, he might seek vengeance against all of you. Even the people of my realm support him. I am from Cedi, but he was born in their kingdom, he is a native Magadhan. In fact the people demanded a festival to honor the Asura sorceress Jarā who saved his life. He is handsome, charming, he has the country on his side. Yet he is a mighty Asura who seeks to control the Earth. I fear him. I feared for *your* lives. I fear for the Earth. Forgive me. I just don't know what I *should* have done, what I *could* have done."

Silence followed these words. Sympathy softened the faces of the younger brothers. No one spoke. The wind blew harder. Sand flew in their faces, high thin trees bent and rocked. Palm fronds shivered. The sea dashed the shore with foaming waves. Then, moody nature grew calm. Vasu's second son spoke.

"I understand," Kuśāmba said to his elder brother. "I'm sure we all understand. When Indra himself could not stop the Asura, how can we blame you? We are all united in purpose and understanding. But now, we must decide what, if anything, we can do to protect our heirs. I understand that the first two generations are not in danger. But the third generation…what can we do? My dear brothers, we must find a way to protect our children when we are all gone. Our father must know what is best."

All the princes and Satya-vatī turned to face the king. His queen did so as well. Vasu took a deep breath, gazed around at his family, and said, "There are steps we can take. First, and most obvious, we will no longer expand our empire beyond Matsya's new realm. My sons, each of you has a prosperous kingdom to rule. Bṛhad-ratha, for the sake of Earth, and other worlds, you must renounce your dream of ruling the Earth. I know your intention was noble, to unite the world in Dharma, to promote peace and justice and to protect Earth from the Asura invasion. But we see now that no matter what we do, Jarā-sandha will inherit Magadha, and with it a leading position in our Cedi dynasty. Indra himself has decided that by all means, we must prevent Jarā-sandha from inheriting imperial power. Indra's decision is that when I retire to the Final Forest, imperial power will return to the Kurus of Hastinā-pura, now led by Śan-tanu."

The five powerful sons of Vasu sat stunned, their lifelong dreams suddenly gone. Some of them wept, but all saw the absolute need to prevent Jarā-sandha from grasping imperial power over the Earth.

"So as of now," Vasu continued, "we renounce any effort to expand our dynasty, however noble the intention. To build empire now is to feed the Asura's power. All of you will continue to be mighty kings, but our first priority must be to contain the mighty Asura Jarā-sandha."

Everyone sadly agreed, but the problem remained of protecting the third generation of Cedi rulers, the sons of the four younger brothers, from the Asuras, led by Jarā-sandha.

"There too," the king said, "I have a plan. As you know, I was born into the powerful Kuru line. Considering the grave danger we face, you may seek an alliance with the young Kuru king, Śan-tanu. His saintly father, Pratīpa, departed to the Final Forest. Śan-tanu is a faithful son, but quite different from his father. Śan-tanu is a fighter. I know none better. Sages say he came down from the Deva realm to help fight the Asuras. His young son Deva-vrata also came from the Deva world and will be as strong as his father. We cannot stop Jarā-sandha from inheriting Magadha, but we can appeal to Śan-tanu to aid us in protecting the world from the Asuras."

"But Father," Kuśāmba said, "Indra gave you, and presumably your sons, the task of protecting this world."

"Yes, but the mightiest Asura has infiltrated our family. Let us face that fact. We must forget old rivalries and forge an alliance with Śan-tanu. He may be open now to our friendship. His wife, Gaṅgā Devī herself, came down from the Deva world to marry him. But though her sacred waters flow here, she could not tolerate life on Earth. 'Let my sacred waters be my service to Earth,' she said. 'They will purify good souls and give them the power to oppose evil.' She then left Śan-tanu and took their son with her. Apparently that loss devastated Śan-tanu. Now is the time to offer him our friendship. In his sadness, he will appreciate true friends, especially those who share his Kuru blood."

"I agree," Matsya said. "The Asuras will not attack a revitalized Kuru dynasty led by Śan-tanu, and allied with Cedi power."

"But how can we persuade him to fight with us?" Bṛhad-ratha asked. "And if we do, how can we be sure he will not try to dominate us?"

King Vasu listened intently, then said, "We know that Śan-tanu has brought several lands under his protection. He is reasserting, indeed reconstructing, the great Kuru dynasty. To *us* he sends messages that he will never disrespect me or my sons. He will honor our mandate from Indra. But Śan-tanu pointedly refuses to give any assurance to our third generation. He knows Jarā-sandha."

"Don't you see, Father," Bṛhad-ratha said, "that our dynasty will sink? The Kurus are taking control, and you allow them. I was to be emperor after you."

"My son, we have no choice. Śan-tanu came to Earth from the Deva realm. He is powerful. The problem is not how *we* can accept *him*. No, the problem is how we can *persuade* him to ally with us. I sent him messages. He always replies in a most courteous, respectful way. He is a noble king and would never disrespect me. But he resists an alliance. I can tell that he resents us. For centuries, the Kurus were the first of kings. Then as Śan-tanu's retiring father, Pratīpa, looked on, and with the blessings of Indra, I became emperor of the world. Śan-tanu must also know about Jarā-sandha. Thus he has two strong motives to mistrust and avoid us. First, by Indra's command, we took a position that for centuries belonged to the Kurus of Hastinā-pura. And second, our dynasty is destined to fall within the grip of a most dangerous Asura."

"He has every reason to avoid us," Kuśāmba said.

"Every reason but one," Matsya argued. "The Kurus and Cedis need each other. We *must* unite for the good of the three worlds."

"I agree," King Vasu said. "I see no other way for those who will never surrender to the Asuras. But it is not easy to secure Śan-tanu's alliance. He trusts me personally, I am sure, but he knows I will retire soon and he fears Jarā-sandha's influence in our family. I beg you all, do not take offense. Were you in Śan-tanu's place, you would share his feelings."

"Then what can be done?" Satya-vatī asked.

"We must wait for now," Vasu said. "Indra knows that our family has been compromised by the birth of Jarā-sandha. Indra may have no choice but to empower young Śan-tanu. Fortunately, Śan-tanu is devoted to Viṣṇu, who has not come yet."

"Then surely Viṣṇu will bring our two families together!" Satya-vatī said, seeing a ray of hope in Śan-tanu's devotion to Viṣṇu.

Everyone looked at her with surprise and appreciation. "You really do have confidence in Viṣṇu," Matsya said.

"Of course," Satya said. "Viṣṇu sent Dvaipāyana to this world, so he must care about us. Surely, you all believe that."

Everyone did believe it. Still, Satya saw that her simple, strong faith, nourished in a country village, startled her sophisticated royal family. But she also saw admiration in their eyes and expressions.

"Well," Matsya said, "we seem to agree that Viṣṇu will somehow unite the Kurus and Cedis. We do have an Avatāra in the family, and I'm sure *he* will help. Satya did tell us that her son promised to help her in her hour of need. Isn't that right Satya?"

"Yes, well, he said that if I needed him, he would quickly come."

"I'm satisfied with that," Matsya said. "Saving Earth must qualify as a legitimate need." He glanced at his twin and raised his eyebrows, as if asking for confirmation of his thesis. Satya nodded and smiled.

"Finally," King Vasu said, "all my sons must continue to fight at all costs to defend Viṣṇu's brāhmaṇas. The Asuras are now proceeding cautiously, killing small numbers of brāhmaṇas in remote places, as we saw near Satya's village. As we know, the Asuras believe they are slowly weakening Viṣṇu. They are sure that Viṣṇu will not descend to this world. Or that if he does he will be sufficiently weakened that the Asuras will slay him. We reject that idea. But you must, I beg you all, protect the sages."

This most sobering report left the entire family silent. Everyone grieved for the sages. Satya-vatī remembered the sage who was like a loving grandfather, till the Asuras killed him.

Queen Girikā now spoke. "There is a most important family matter that we must resolve. "Where will dear Satya live?"

"She will live in my kingdom," Matsya said.

"That would be an excellent plan," Bṛhad-ratha said, "and I dearly wish she could go there. But Matsya came to realize that Jarā-sandha suspected Satya-vatī from the moment he saw her in the palace gardens. And he clearly knows that Satya came with us today on the crystal aircraft, while he was left behind. I'm truly sorry, Satya, but it would be unwise for you to live in any of our realms, at least for now. Jarā-sandha is too dangerous. We feel his pressure on our minds. Indeed a short time ago, right after he met Satya-vatī, Jarā-sandha asked my permission to stay here in Cedi when I return to Magadha. He said he wanted time with his grandparents, but in fact he assumed that Satya would be here. I could not refuse his request without increasing his suspicion."

"What are you saying?" Matsya exclaimed.

"I am saying this," replied Bṛhad-ratha. "If Satya goes to your realm, Matsya, you will have to explain why you treat her like your sister. What will you say? I have no doubt that my son has allies and spies throughout our kingdoms. He will monitor her presence there. If Satya-vatī goes with you, Jarā-sandha will discover a strong desire to visit you. It is likely that he already knows about the Avatāra. How will you refuse your own nephew the right to visit you? That would fully arouse his suspicion. No, let us be clear. If Satya goes to your realm, Matsya, Jarā-sandha will follow her there. And he will find a most discreet way to place Satya in danger and so force the Avatāra to come to her rescue. Naturally, it will be a trap to kill the Avatāra."

"Oh, heaven forbid!" Satya-vatī cried.

"Exactly," Bṛhad-ratha said. "Heaven does forbid it and thus we cannot unwittingly enable such an evil. Therefore, most sadly I say that Satya must even leave Cedi as quickly as possible. As awful as it sounds, we have no choice but to ask Satya to remain concealed for a little while longer till the Avatāra has developed his full powers."

Matsya now spoke up, facing his eldest brother. "But our father just told us that Jarā-sandha will not give us any good reason to deny him his inheritance. So how could he plot to kill the Avatāra in one of our kingdoms?"

"What Father said is true," Bṛhad-ratha replied. "My so-called son does not wish to jeopardize his legitimate inheritance. That is why I tried to make clear that he will engineer his plot so that no evidence can be brought against him. But make no mistake, he will not pass up a chance to slay a young Avatāra who may not yet possess all his powers."

Seeing Satya-vatī fearful and crestfallen, Kuśāmba said, "My dear sister, when your son develops his full powers, which will be soon, no Asura can harm him. And at the first possible opportunity, we shall all welcome you into our kingdoms with the genuine love of most devoted brothers. You will be honored and adored as you deserve."

Satya-vatī thanked him with real affection, and said, "Sadly, I must agree."

Queen Girikā then said, "Regarding my beloved daughter, there is a further point. For her own happiness and safety, Satya must marry. And she must marry at her own level. She is a princess. But what prince will marry a girl who is known to have given birth out of wedlock? Of course, we can say that her son was an Avatāra, and that is true. But Avatāra Dvaipāyana may not reveal himself to the world for several years. So who would believe us? How will Satya convince the world of her divine mission? And the many Asuras who now infiltrate so many kingdoms, including ours, will slander her and make very sure that no worthy prince seeks her hand. So as terrible as it sounds, I advise that for now, our beloved daughter continue to conceal her identity."

"It breaks my heart," King Vasu said, "but I must agree with your mother. Satya is beautiful and she is my daughter. Many princes will vie for her hand. But they will not accept that she had a child before marriage, even if Viṣṇu himself arranged to send her an Avatāra. We live in a cruel world and we must act wisely. And for now, we must conceal the Avatāra's birth. That means we have no way to explain Satya-vatī's long separation from her family. It will all work out for the best, I know. I ask you to trust me and your mother here."

Satya-vatī felt her heart breaking, but she found no flaw in her family's logic. For now, she could not openly live with her family. The public would continue to see her as the daughter of a fishing family. But the thought of returning to her village oppressed her exceedingly. She could not return there now, no matter what anyone said. But where could she go? Her mother was speaking and she must pay attention. Her thoughts about herself must wait.

"My dear children," Queen Girikā said, "your father and I have done all we could to protect this planet, but the time has come for us to retire. We have been telling you this for some time. Now we must formally declare it. We shall now hand over all power to our sons and retire to the Final Forest. There, we will prepare for our journey to the World Beyond. You will all be safe for now. The Avatāra will also be safe."

Satya-vatī and her five brothers sat motionless. She had just been reunited with her parents and now they were abandoning her again.

"Must you really retire now?" their fourth son, Pratyagra asked. "It is too soon."

"I have no wish to abandon you," the king said, "but your time has come. My time has ended. We must all obey the will of Providence. Indra did not, indeed, he *cannot*, grant eternal life in a material body. Only Viṣṇu may grant full immortality. It is now the time ordained for your mother and me to retire to the Final Forest. That is why we called you all here."

Cries of protest against this idea rose from his children, but the king simply shook his head and looked kindly on his family. "Now, you my sons must protect the world."

The queen then said, "We discussed where my beloved daughter, Satya-vatī, would go. Of course she is free to choose, but your father and I want very much that she come with us. Just the three of us. It is our greatest wish to spend our last year on Earth with Satya-vatī."

These words sent a thrill through Satya's heart.

"Dear girl," the king said, "we will not force you if your heart is set on something else, but if you are willing to come with us, just for a year, nothing could make us happier."

Nothing could have made Satya happier and with all her feeling, she agreed and embraced her parents. She remembered what Parā-śara said about a future marriage, but that would come in time. She seized this last chance to live with her parents.

In all this joy, questions troubled her. Would the world be safe without her father to protect it? Would her brothers be safe? Could her son, the Avatāra, protect himself from the Asuras, who would surely grow bolder now that the emperor retired? Would Viṣṇu come? Could Viṣṇu himself defeat the Asuras?

CHAPTER 17

The day before Satya-vatī's departure with her parents, the royal family went to the crystal aircraft to bid it farewell. It would return to Indra's world.

Matsya told Satya, "Indra only allowed our father to control it. We do not have our father's mental strength. We did not practice severe yoga as he did for many years. Also, Indra feared the craft might fall into Jarā-sandha's hands. Bṛhad-ratha always dreamed of flying that aircraft. But we will all do our best. I just hope that Śan-tanu will come to his senses and form an alliance with us. He is always polite, but will not enter a formal alliance. That is my main concern. Anyway, don't worry about all that. Enjoy your time with our parents."

As the royal family stood at attention, the aircraft rose slowly into the air, hovered above them, and vanished from view, rushing through inner space back to Indra's world. Vasu recounted how the crystal aircraft first appeared to him and Girikā, how they took their first flight together, and how the aircraft empowered him to save many sages, and to defeat many Asuras.

The family walked slowly back to the palace. That night, their last in Pearl River, Girikā took Satya in one hand, the king in the other, and eagerly pulled them to a palace balcony that overlooked the river. She pointed out the exact spot where the king rescued her when he first arrived in Cedi. Aware that Parāśara had revealed the scene to Satya-vatī, the queen spoke to her daughter in animated tones about the king's daring rescue. Vasu smiled and thanked Indra and Viṣṇu.

That evening, Matsya spent as much time as possible with his twin, promising to visit her and his parents often in the Final Forest.

Satya bid all her brothers farewell that night, for in the next day's departure ceremony, she must pretend to be a mere attendant to the royal couple. She slept in the palace.

The morning came. Countless citizens of town and country came to bid their king and queen farewell. Women and men wept openly. Most had never known another ruler. All the citizens looked upon King Vasu and Queen Girikā as loving parents who always protected and cared for them. Born in Pearl River, Girikā had loved her citizens from childhood, and they loved her.

Through a trusted courier, Satya-vatī informed her foster parents that she had accepted an invitation to attend to the king and queen in the Final Forest, till they departed for the World Beyond. After that, she would visit them. Satya knew her fosters parents would not come to the departure ceremony. They never traveled.

In a solemn but colorful ceremony, in the grand plaza of the royal palace, Vasu and Girikā sat with government and military leaders, as representatives from all social classes bid moving farewells to their king and queen. Then the five sons, dressed in the royal garb, visibly struggling to control their emotions, offered eloquent praise to their parents.

Finally, senior brāhmaṇas, many of whom owed their lives to the king, chanted prayers from the Veda and offered heartfelt thanks and blessings to the royal couple. They knew that their king and queen would never have hesitated to give their lives for them.

A royal band, dressed smartly in colorful uniforms, played the Cedi anthem. This concluded the farewell ceremony.

The king and queen, with their five sons, and a daughter disguised as a royal attendant, accompanied by an elite palace guard, rolled out of the city in three open carriages, pulled smoothly by high-stepping horses. They headed for the Final Forest, a full day's journey away.

Thousands of citizens followed the carriages, till they reached a narrow bridge over the Pearl River. Here the king thanked his people for the last time, and prayed for their eternal well-being. As the three carriages with their military escort crossed the bridge in single file, soldiers quickly closed in behind them, sealing the bridge. The king and his party proceeded alone to the Final Forest.

Satya-vatī rode with her parents. As they crossed the bridge, she looked back and saw Jarā-sandha. His face revealed his mind. He was silently celebrating the king's departure. He must know that none of the king's sons could match their father's power. The Asura turned to her with a smile that sent shivers up her spine. She prayed to Viṣṇu to protect her brothers, and turned her gaze back to the forward path.

The mood on the journey was serious, though many affectionate words and smiles were exchanged between Satya and her parents. She still yearned for a loving marriage, but cherished this chance to assist her parents in their final days, just as much as they longed for her company. All three were determined to make up for lost time.

Absorbed in her thoughts, Satya was brought to attention by a sudden jarring that shook the carriage. They had turned off the main road and now traveled on a rough trail that traversed a deep forest with towering trees. All villages and farms were left behind. The carriage stopped, for the other two carriages, carrying her brothers and royal guards now turned back. With waves and tears, they bid each other farewell. Satya-vatī and her parents moved alone toward the Final Forest.

The forest grew larger and denser, at times abruptly opening to reveal virgin green meadows that shimmered with ponds and lakes. The ambience was so idyllic that Satya-vatī wanted to cry out in joy. Even the carriage's jolting made her feel like a child being rocked in its mother's arms.

At last, the horses stopped. The journey ended. Satya wanted to look around at the place that would be her home for at least a year. But a group of elderly brāhmaṇas, husbands and wives, hurried to the carriage and welcomed them. Greetings on both sides were so warm and familiar that Satya understood that these were old and intimate acquaintances. Her parents introduced Satya to the sages as a beloved friend of the family that had kindly come from another land to take care of them during their time here. The sages greeted her warmly, but showed no interest in further kinship details, and the king and queen had no inclination to explain further.

Satya saw that her parents had chosen well the sages who would guide them in their last days. These brāhmaṇas were longtime trusted friends of the royal couple, yet they knew enough of royal affairs not to inquire about the details of the ruler's personal life. Here was a perfect balance of intimacy and reserve, familiarity and discretion.

The sages led the king and queen to a simple but comfortable hut. Like everything else here, it was immaculate. The neighboring hut was for Satya. She felt perfectly comfortable here and gave heartfelt thanks to her saintly hosts.

The brāhmaṇa ladies invited the queen and Satya to bathe in the nearby river in a private area and they happily agreed. Queen Girikā playfully grabbed Satya's hand and led her down to the riverbank. After their ablutions, they dressed in the spotless white cloth used in the Final Forest. Girikā explained to her daughter that these sages were Vaikhānasas, an ancient brāhmaṇa community that served as guides for retiring couples. "In every kingdom," she said, "there is a Final Forest, and these sages guide those who seek to perfect their spiritual consciousness in the final stage of life. They will teach us where to find pure drinking water, what forest fruits and plants to eat, how to stay warm, how to avoid dangerous animals and insects — in short, how to live in the Final Forest."

"These Vaikhānasa sages are certainly very kind and expert," Satya said.

"Yes, and even more important, they will guide us spiritually so that when we leave Earth, we will attain our chosen world."

"Mother, tell me what world you and Father chose for your next life. I want to join you there when I leave Earth. You and Father have a special relationship with Indra and his wife, Śacī. Will you go to their world?"

"Oh no, my dear. We are most grateful to Indra and Śacī, as they well know. But even in their Deva world, everyone dies eventually, even Indra, though they enjoy a fabulous lifespan. No, your father and I do not seek to enjoy any world in this universe. We want only to serve Viṣṇu's mission. He will strategically place us where we are most needed. If he so commands us, we will return to this world. Our ultimate goal, once our duties are done in this universe, is the World Beyond, Viṣṇu's world. Only there is life everlasting."

Satya smiled at the thought of living forever in Viṣṇu's world, with all those whom she loved. Her father smiled and said, "My dear girl, if you like, let us explore our new home."

"Most gladly!" Satya said, proud of her parents' devotion. Taking her father's hand, she set off to walk about the Vaikhānasa campus.

It was a large settlement encompassing various residential areas. There were convenient bathing areas, simple cooking facilities, with dining areas consisting of straw sitting mats, and banana-leaf plates.

Satya and her parents saw arenas for fire sacrifice. In other areas, sages recited mantras and taught sacred texts to those who wished to learn. Girikā joined them as they came upon a space reserved for serious yoga meditation. Vasu smiled. "I think I can still do it."

"Really?" Girikā replied. "Then you must teach me. As a girl, I used to dream of becoming a yoginī, if no handsome prince married me. But he did."

Satya-vatī was happy to see that her parents, having given up the burden of governance, were joyfully, youthfully, embracing their new life. And now Satya herself would have a chance to live the life of the saintly sages she had served and loved since her early childhood! The Final Forest reminded her of the brāhmaṇa community on the Yamunā, across from her village.

At first, the austere life in the Final Forest was easier for Satya-vatī, who had always lived a simple life. But her parents quickly adapted. When Satya saw her parents dressed in white robes, she recalled her vision of young Prince Vasu as a yogī, even before he met Lord Indra, before he met Girikā and became emperor.

Satya was proud of her parents. She understood more and more that they had truly engaged power and opulence as a service to the world, and to Viṣṇu. And now, after so many adventures and battles, they had happily embraced an intense spiritual path.

They were given ample free time, and one day, her father told her, "Dear girl, your mother and I are about to enter lengthy meditation. But before that, I thought, only if you like the idea, that I could teach you to ride a horse."

"A horse? Really?"

"Yes, my dear. Perhaps it's just the wish of a foolish old man."

"My dear father, you're not old; you're just retired."

The emperor laughed. "Thank you, my dear. I would have most happily taught you that, had I been blessed to raise you. Perhaps now we can capture at least a little of the happiness we missed. You've grown into such a beautiful, brilliant young lady. If you like, we could do that together now."

Satya agreed with such joy that she could hardly contain her laughs and tears. For the next few days, father and daughter rode about the surrounding forests. Satya quickly learned to ride well, and on their last day riding, they went deep into the forest, and talked for hours, revealing their hearts to each other. It was a moment Satya-vatī would never forget.

She would sit near her parents for yoga practice. She regularly glanced at them. At every moment she felt grateful to Viṣṇu in her heart. Satya-vatī had never been happier, never more carefree. Vasu eagerly returned to the yoga practice of his youth and Girikā joined him, in every way his equal in spiritual discipline.

Then Satya-vatī saw something amazing. As her parents entered deeply into their spiritual meditation, they seemed to regain all the beauty and vigor of their youth. They looked just as they did when, by the mercy of Parā-śara, Satya first saw them falling in love, after Vasu rescued Girikā from the river flood.

The family heard daily classes from learned sages who explained how by transcending attachment to the body and its possessions, one frees the pure soul.

Life went on steadily for a few months in the Final Forest. Satya's parents felt increasingly comfortable and peaceful in their new life, missing only their sons. Then one day, Bṛhad-ratha and Matsya came to see their parents and sister.

Anxious not to disturb the other practitioners, the brothers camped right outside the Final Forest, and visited daily, wearing simple dress, leaving their weapons with their guards and attendants. The first day, the brothers avoided any worldly topic, eagerly inquiring from their parents about their comfort, progress in self-realization, and hopes for ultimate liberation. They were relieved and gratified by the answers they received.

But on the second day, the brothers made many apologies and then asked if they could seek advice from their father on worldly matters. Vasu could not refuse them. Girikā and Satya-vatī took part in the family talk.

The brothers revealed that with the crystal aircraft gone, armies loyal to the Devas were placed on a state of heightened alert. Śan-tanu, Bṛhad-ratha, and other strong monarchs increasingly offered help to less powerful kingdoms, and to some extent vied for alliances with strategically important kingdoms. There was an increase of Asura attacks in some remote locations. Brāhmaṇas loyal to Viṣṇu now avoided certain areas.

These events were distressing, but did not tip the global balance of power. The Cedi kings continued to hope that Śan-tanu would see the advantages of a Cedi alliance. Bṛhad-ratha lamented the slow, steady shift of political and military leadership to Śan-tanu. But he knew that imperial power could never pass to his Asura son, Jarā-sandha.

"Indeed," he said, "Jarā-sandha watches this shift of power to the Kurus with growing resentment. He was desperate to inherit supreme power when I am gone. But now he sees the rise of Śan-tanu and the growing restoration of Kuru supremacy and it angers him. God only knows what he will do when I am gone. But forgive me, Father, I should not have mentioned this."

Vasu listened to his son sympathetically, but made few comments. Matsya then said, "I dearly wish that I had better news to report, but instead, I have just heard from diplomatic sources that Gaṅgā Devī brought back to Śan-tanu their powerful young son Deva-vrata. Śan-tanu deeply laments the loss of Gaṅgā, but with a demigod son at his side, he must believe more than ever that he does not need a Cedi alliance to defend the world."

Satya and her family were convinced that Śan-tanu was tragically mistaken. But no one could convince that headstrong young warrior whose power steadily increased.

"He does not understand Asura power," Matsya lamented. "He underestimates it, and this mistake will lead to tragedy for him and the world. If only he could understand."

Seeing how much the stubborn Kuru lord Śan-tanu disturbed her parents in their final days on Earth, Satya-vatī felt increasing anger and resentment toward him. "Why is he so foolish?" she asked her mother.

"My dear," the queen said, "we don't fully understand Śan-tanu. I hesitate to judge him at this point, though I wish as much as anyone that he would work with us."

"I believe that Śan-tanu must be very proud indeed," Satya said.

"He may be," Girikā said. "He is fairly young, handsome, from what we hear, and he rules the great Kuru realm. He may be a good man at heart. If only one of us could speak openly and sincerely with him. But he avoids us."

"Sadly, I do not believe he is a good man," Satya said. "But time will tell."

The next day, Bṛhad-ratha and Matsya departed. Satya-vatī was thrilled to see them, and sad to see them go, but she understood the gravity of their duties. Her other three brothers visited soon after, but did not raise political issues with their parents.

As time passed, Satya-vatī felt as if she had never been separated from her parents. Their love for each other was as strong as Satya could wish. In fact, her parents thought of her comfort so much that she had to remind them to pay attention to their yoga practice.

A year passed and the day came for Vasu and Girikā to depart. They happily placed their fate fully in Viṣṇu's hands. Lord Indra and Śacī Devī appeared within the couple's meditation and bid them farewell. Vasu thanked his Deva patrons wholeheartedly for all they had done, and wished them success in their battle with the Asuras.

It was most difficult for Vasu and Girikā to bid farewell to their daughter. "We will await you in Viṣṇu's world," they told her, "when your duties here are done."

In the presence of Satya-vatī and all the gathered sages, Vasu and Girikā sat in deep, final meditation. Satya-vatī watched intensely till she saw their glowing souls rise steadily from one bodily cakra to another, till they departed the body and entered into spiritual space.

Young brāhmaṇas came and took the empty bodies to the funeral pyre for the last rites. Satya knew that Viṣṇu had personally taken her parents and she rejoiced as she wept.

The last rites came and went, but Satya's heart and mind could not focus on them. Heavy thoughts, feelings, and visions filled her mind. Remembrances of one duty steadied her. She would keep her promise to visit her foster parents. How much had changed since she left her village in a little boat, determined to escape her chaperones at the first opportunity! How much she herself had changed!

When her parents departed, Satya-vatī wished to leave at once. She had to keep busy to stop her mind from falling prey to grief. She sent word to her brothers, but had no patience to wait for them to arrange her passage back to her village. So, after taking proper leave of the sages of the Final Forest, with many heartfelt thanks, Satya-vatī left on the next carriage that arrived bringing pious, elderly persons there.

Her parents and brothers had given her very generous gifts, and she need only ask to receive more. Though she must hide it from the world, she was now, at eighteen, an extremely wealthy young woman. Her material needs would never be a problem.

As she bounced down the narrow road that led to the highway, she reflected on her life. On the sad side, her own son, Dvaipāyana, was denied to her, and for now, she could not spend much time with her brothers.

For now, at least, she would return to the humble and humbling village where she grew up. All her birth family were lost to her till she married a prince or king who could guarantee her safety, or until her Avatāra son had fully realized his powers and was safe from any Asura attack.

Despite her grief, worries, and conjectures, Satya-vatī was strong at heart, convinced that all these events had a higher purpose. Parā-śara assured her of that, and she preferred to believe him. For the general future, Satya's heart was set on a happy marriage. Her Avatāra son would come instantly if ever she really needed him. But she would not engage an Avatāra as her matchmaker. For now, she would soldier on alone, and wait for better times that would surely come.

The carriage was heading south and Satya was going north, so at the first town, she hired a private conveyance. She again preferred to travel alone. She had so much on her mind, she could not bear an unwanted companion. She stopped briefly in the village where she left her little boat and paid a small sum to have it rowed upstream back to her village. She was too weak with emotion, and from the austerities of the Final Forest, to steer a small boat so far.

The pain she felt at her parents' departure mixed with the joy of her precious time with them. Inspired by their love for her, she breathed a new confidence. She knew, with serene determination, that for the rest of her life, she would strive to make them proud of her. She had five loving brothers, and a happy future promised by Parā-śara.

Despite all the blessings that buoyed her, pain at the loss of parents so recently found must still afflict her. But it could not confuse or defeat her. Even that pain now inspired her to live a life that would please her parents, and make them proud. With all these and more feelings, she set out into the world. She was a king's daughter, and she began to make necessary calculations.

Satya could have taken a boat down Pearl River. It would pass through the Cedi capital and continue northeast toward the Yamunā and her village. Instead, she had chosen to bypass the capital. She craved solitude.

Satya-vatī's brothers had told her they had secret agents throughout Cedi and other countries, and that they would track her for her safety. Jarā-sandha vaguely suspected her and probably ordered that she be watched by ubiquitous Asura agents.

The Kurus fielded a vast network of agents. They probably did not know her real identity, but she had intimately served great Vasu and his wife. The Kurus would assume that the royal couple might have revealed this or that state secret to a devoted girl attending them in their final days. Thus by the same logic of the Asuras, that Satya-vatī could possess valuable information, the Kurus must have also decided that she was entitled to surveillance.

Making her way toward her village, passing all varieties of people, she wondered how many faces, from how many lands, were trailing and watching her.

CHAPTER 18

Riding in a private carriage, on decent roads, Satya-vatī safely approached her village in Kalpi. A mile from the village, she saw a familiar middle-aged couple. It was the kind fishing couple that was supposed to serve as chaperones on her first trip to Śukti-matī, the Cedi capital.

Drawing closer, she leaned out the carriage window, called to them, and waved. They smiled, called back, and hurried over to the carriage window. The lady squeezed her arm, and the man gave a little bow. They apologized for losing her on the trip, though the quick glance the couple exchanged told the real story. They knew that Satya had escaped from them. But they were too polite to say that to the village chief's daughter.

The lady looked at her and looked again. Her expression changed, because Satya had changed. She was dressed well. Nothing of finery or ostentation, but she was dressed like a lady from the Cedi capital. Her hair was properly combed.

Satya no longer had the will or patience to speak like a fishing girl, and that was another problem. Or at least another big surprise for her old acquaintances, who had never heard the fine speech she formerly reserved for the brāhmaṇa village across the river.

All in all, the kindly couple both knew and didn't know Satya-vatī, and this so confused them that they simply said nice things and waved her on since her parents must be so anxious to see her.

This brief meeting outside the village was but a harbinger of worse things to come inside the village. First, though merely respectable in the capital, the carriage turned heads in Kalpi. Indeed, such a fine carriage had never before rolled into the muddy, malodorous fishing village. That it carried a fishing girl from Kalpi, even the fisher king's daughter, made it a startling event that would be talked of for much time to come.

When the villagers saw and heard the transformation in Satya-vatī — her dress, speech, and manner — they all stared agape. Of course, everyone knew that Satya-vatī had faithfully served the emperor and empress, but this only increased their wonder and wide-eyed stares. Hearing of their daughter's return, Dāśa-rāja and his wife hurried to the scene as quickly as their dignity would allow.

Most uneasy of all was Satya-vatī. On the way "home," she had unwisely allowed feelings of guilt and nostalgia to filter and color her memories and expectations of the village and its people. Within a few moments of her entrance there, indeed moments before that, she had realized that she could never, ever, live in that village again.

For the moment, she played her part well. She greeted, smiled at, and embraced all the right people at all the right moments. That night, alone in her cottage, trying to sleep after a tiring trip, she could not stop crying. It pained her to offend these people, especially her foster parents, but she could not live like them.

This was not her home. She had no home in the world, no place to rest her mind and soul. She would go mad if she stayed here. Finally, she slept for a few hours.

Seeing how tired she looked on her arrival, though not knowing that she was still grieving the loss of her real parents, Dāśa-rāja and his wife did not ask about her time away until the next day, when she appeared to be more rested. They all sat down together for breakfast. Her foster father treated her with love tinged by resentment, and her foster mother showed concern bordering on alarm.

Satya had no strength to conceal her deep transformation. Dāśa-rāja and his wife saw in her face and manner, indeed in every word, look, and gesture, that she was almost a different person.

Dāśa-rāṇi, the woman Satya-vatī had always loved as her mother, trembled, and said in a miserable voice, "What did they tell you in the great capital? Did they say anything about your father and me? About who your parents are? Is that why you stayed away so long?"

What could Satya say? She considered telling a white lie. No! That was absurd. These simple, hard-working people, who had loved her, in their way, all her life, would see through it at once, and that would make things worse. Satya braced her heart and said, "I learned that I was born in the Cedi capital, to other parents, and for some reason, I was sent to you. Is that true?"

Tears streamed down Dāśa-rāṇi's face. "Yes, it is true. We wanted to tell you, but they forbade us. Who told you? They didn't let us tell you and now someone else did. Satya, don't blame us. They didn't let us tell you. But we always loved you as a daughter. Maybe you don't love us anymore."

Satya-vatī rushed to her and embraced her tightly, vowing her love for the humble fisherwoman who had devotedly raised her. Dāśa-rāja looked on quietly, pensively. When the two women turned to him, he said, "You may wonder, dear girl, why we never visited you in the great capital."

"I know you don't like to travel," she said.

"That is true," the burly man said.

What could any one of them say? Satya-vatī assured them of her love and could do no more. In the following days, she tried her best to behave like their daughter. It was a trial that taxed her piety.

Life in Śukti-matī, an ecstatic reunion with her birth family, the priceless time spent caring for her exalted parents in their last days, the love she received from everyone in her royal family, people who actually understood her, and loved her for who she really was, all that had transformed her beyond return.

As the days passed, the pressure to engage in constant theater, with endless dissembling and pretense, wore down her spirits. Satya-vatī sank into a listless fog of depression.

She could not shed a royal reserve and dignity that bewildered her foster parents, and convinced the other villagers that the great capital had spoiled her and made her forget who she was. Most disturbing was the resentment of a proud foster father who found it hard to truly forgive her for choosing to serve another family, even if it was the imperial family of Cedi. Never directly, but with a word here, a hint there, he revealed a deep resentment.

Beyond this, her foster parents did not trouble her. After long separation, neither side wanted to provoke the other. They exchanged embraces, avoided open confrontation, and pretended on both sides that all was fine.

How long her foster parents could pretend would not be tested. Satya-vatī could not bear to continue playing the part of a fishing girl. She would rather give herself up to goddess Yamunā and drown in her waters.

But that too was not a serious option, not when she carried within her heart Parā-śara's solemn assurance of future happiness; not when she still cherished the hope of helping her brothers; and certainly not while her Avatāra son still lived, and she had the power to summon him someday.

She might have spent time happily in the brāhmaṇa village across the river, but it was a community of all elder men. To live in a hamlet where she had only made day visits her entire life would confuse both sides of the river, and likely create friction.

After brooding for days over a course of action, she saw that her only present option was to seek solitude on Yamunā's waters and in the great forests she knew so well. She informed her foster parents of her intention to spend some time alone. She spoke with such dignified determination — and so consistent was this declaration with all of her behavior since returning — that after a gentle protest, which they saw as their duty, they shrugged their shoulders and said, "You are grown now. What can we do? After all we've done for you, if you love us at all, be careful and stay safe. And come back soon."

Satya-vatī assured them of her love for them, spoke her undying gratitude for all they had done, and promised she would avoid danger. She would visit them soon. "I will just be going down the river a bit. If someone needs me, they can find me on the river, or near it, close to the shore." She said this in case her brothers or Parā-śara happened to look for her, or send a message.

After saying many nice things to ease her departure, Satya put her few belongings in a bag, and ran to her boat. She placed a few drops of sacred river water on her head and bowed to Yamunā, praying to be protected on her journey.

Setting off, she first crossed to the brāhmaṇa village to beg the blessings of the sages. The sages eagerly blessed her. She thanked and honored them with deep affection.

After pushing off in her boat, she floated downstream to the southeast. If she continued in this direction for many days, Yamunā would merge into the Gaṅgā. She realized with astonishment that Śan-tanu had actually married the goddess of that famous river. No wonder he was so insufferably proud. And no wonder goddess Gaṅgā left him. Satya-vatī would not travel that far.

On the first day, as the sun sank into the river, she stopped after a few hours. Tying her boat on the north shore, she set up camp, using the survival skills she learned in the Final Forest.

The next day, she rose early and set off to explore the forest that was alive with bright, singing birds, and rich with ripened fruits and herbs. In the afternoon, she rested in her camp and meditated on her life. After a few days of this routine, she was bored.

Eager for change, for hope, she moved eastward toward Yamunā's confluence with the Kena River. Weeks passed. At times she stopped at riverside villages, at times in wilderness, or in meadows and fields, always near the riverbank.

A message came from Bṛhad-ratha, via one of his most trusted royal couriers. Satya had told her brothers she would visit her foster parents. The courier first went to their village and was told to head down the Yamunā till he found her, which he did. Satya-vatī had not seen Bṛhad-ratha since his last visit to the Final Forest.

The message was this:

"My dear sister, we are all well, but that is all the encouraging news we have. On the political front, I regret to tell you that my 'son' Jarā-sandha continues to grow stronger, as does his support from the citizens and even other rulers, who may be Asuras. More of Viṣṇu's brāhmaṇas have been slain, but, thank God, not many, and not in our realm. I have sent gracious messages to proud King Śan-tanu, but he sends back curt replies that leave no room to discuss an alliance. He has no concern for us, though he retains all the polite language of empty diplomacy. He is our own cousin, since our father was a Kuru, but that means nothing to him. I am sorry to tell you all this, but dear Satya-vatī, you are an intimate family member, and I feel you have a right to know all that is happening with us. We value your advice. Dear sister, we deeply regret that you must still conceal your identity, but we know that will change, and hopefully soon. Please, if you need anything at all, grant us the joy of serving you. We all send our love. Your brother, Bṛhad-ratha."

Deeply moved, Satya-vatī sat down by the river to sort out all the thoughts and feelings that this message aroused. Her eldest brother's resolve that she be treated as an intimate and equal family member, and the eager concern of all her brothers to care for her needs, gave deep satisfaction. She rejoiced in her family's complete and loving acceptance.

The other news left her with very different feelings. Jarā-sandha's growing strength caused much concern. And the continued killing of brāhmaṇas brought her to tears.

King Śan-tanu's steady intransigence roused her almost to fury. He was their cousin! One could expect nothing good from a hardened Asura. But one had every right to expect far more from Śan-tanu. The political and military situation depressed her more than her personal problems. Indeed, she forgot them in her grief for her family and the world they were sworn to protect.

That night, these worries troubled her sleep, and in the morning, she went for a long walk to ponder her course of action. In a grassy clearing, she saw a stray horse too far from any village or settlement to have an owner. It was not wild, but had no saddle or blanket. Satya recalled with a smile that when she first met Matsya, he wanted her to ride his horse. Then, her father taught her to ride. Matsya would be amused to hear that she mounted and rode this stray horse, even for a few moments.

The horse seemed friendly enough and ate grass from her hand. Encouraged and fearless, she mounted the horse and patted its neck. The horse took a few steps. That was enough for her. She was about to dismount when the horse suddenly broke into a gallop, racing over the meadow. It stopped suddenly. Satya went flying into a tree. To her horror, she hit it hard. She fell to the ground, unconscious.

CHAPTER 19

Satya-vatī woke up in a darkening dusk. She found herself lying on a blanket. She found the strength to sit up and was shocked to see a large man tending a fire nearby. She must have been seriously injured in the fall, yet she felt no pain. Watching the man, she touched her head and body and found no sign of injury. Thank God! But who is that man? Near him stood a large sword, leaning against a tree. Recalling the hunters who threatened her on the road to Pearl River, she struggled to her feet and grabbed a stick.

He glanced at her and laughed. It was an amused, friendly laugh. It did not seem threatening. But who was he?

"You fell from your horse," he said. "Or perhaps I should say, you fell from *my* horse."

She saw the same horse was grazing nearby. "I waited," he said, "to make sure you're all right. It gets cold here in the evening, so I lit a fire."

"Thank you, sir, for coming to my aid. I do know this area and its weather quite well. I apologize for riding your horse. I thought it was a stray and mounted it for but a moment. But it took off in a gallop and threw me into a tree."

"Yes, he does that when a stranger mounts him. I'm just glad you're all right."

"Again, I thank you, sir. It was kind of you to wait to see if I was injured. I assure you I am not. So, you have done your duty. Fully."

She tried to make it clear that he should leave now. Why did he stay? What were his motives?

"Well, I'm glad to hear that," he said, walking toward her.

"Stay where you are!" She raised her stick. "I do not know you. I mean no offense, but we are not acquainted."

"You're perfectly right," he said, looking amused. "Forgive my informality. On my honor, I mean you no harm. I am Sau-nandya, a traveler from the north. I came to the woods hoping to find peace."

"I hope you find the peace you seek," Satya said. He did not look like a rough or vulgar man. He was large and very strongly built. His manners and speech were those of a gentleman, but his dress showed him to be from common, though respectable, circumstances.

The fire flashed and she saw his face clearly. He was handsome. He was older than her, perhaps ten years or more, but still youthful. She would not reciprocate and give him her name. He might falsely take it as some sort of interest on her part. That would be dangerous.

"Sir," she said, resolved to be explicit, "either you must leave, or if you prefer to stay with the fire, I shall be on my way."

"I will leave at once if you command me, but I do not recommend that you wander alone in these woods."

"And why is that?" she asked.

"It may not be safe. I have heard rumors that Asuras have come to our world, some as wild animals."

"How do you know that?" she demanded, fearing he must be an Asura. After all, few people on Earth knew of the Asura invasion.

"I know because I heard it from Viṣṇu's sages."

Why would Viṣṇu's sages reveal this most secret knowledge to a commoner? This heightened Satya's suspicion. She decided to test him, preparing herself to dash into the woods if he was an Asura. He was far stronger, but she was quick and agile, and knew these forests well.

Asuras were too proud to feign devotion to Viṣṇu, so she asked him, "What do you think of Viṣṇu?"

He did not hesitate. "Viṣṇu is the source of all Avatāras. I serve Viṣṇu alone. That is my vow."

Satya stared at him, unable to shake her incredulity. He smiled. "I see you do not trust me. I understand. In these times, it is best to be extremely cautious. Anyway, I will go and leave you the fire."

The man said this, but he did not leave.

"Sir," Satya-vatī said, "you are staring at me."

The man smiled. "Forgive me, but there's a certain brightness about you. You almost seem to glow."

"Whether I glow or not," Satya-vatī said, "I now wish to be alone."

"Of course," he said, more amused than affronted by her words. He walked to his horse, then turned around and said, "I am going to hunt for dinner now and I will gladly share it with you, if you like."

Satya-vatī replied gravely, "Sir, these woods are full of nourishing fruits, roots, and grains. There is no need to kill our animal neighbors. I mean you no offense, but since there are no dangerous beasts in this forest, assuming the Asuras did not invade here yet, you help no one by killing innocent creatures."

The strong man seemed affronted by these words. But his features quickly softened. He asked with more curiosity than anger, "If I may inquire, who are you to instruct me?"

"I am a soul like you, one who cares about other souls."

The man smiled. "Well spoken. I cannot disagree. And since I am also a soul, you must care about me as well."

"Yes, that is why I spoke to you. With your permission, I will stay here for the evening, and I wish to be alone now. May you also find a suitable place to rest. Goodbye, sir."

"Thank you for your concern. I will trouble you no further. Forgive any impropriety on my part. Good evening, fair lady."

He bowed slightly, mounted his horse, and quickly vanished into the darkening woods. Satya looked on until the dark forest swallowed both sight and sound of the stranger.

She sat by the fire to think and wonder about this chance meeting. Was it wise to stay alone in the great forest, even with the protection of the river goddess? She recollected that her only other option was to return to the fishing village. This sobering thought fixed her resolve to continue her journey, whatever the consequences. Parā-śara had promised future happiness, a loving marriage. Her faith in the sage's words buoyed her. She would continue her odyssey. There was nothing else to do.

The Veda taught that Viṣṇu lives within offering fire. Satya-vatī washed a long, sharp twig in the river, spiked a small grain loaf taken from her bag, and roasted it in the crackling fire. In her heart, she offered this simple food to Viṣṇu and felt his strong, comforting presence in the fire.

The greatest of all Avatāras was now her unseen, but deeply felt, companion. In his presence, Yamunā herself, devoted to Viṣṇu, happily observed Satya-vatī's blessed meal. The little loaf satisfied the Cedi princess. She ate little more than this in her days of high yoga in the Final Forest.

And the curious stranger? She trusted she would never again see that gentleman. She fed the fire, to keep it alive as long as possible, and lay down to rest, trusting that Viṣṇu would protect her from any malevolent creature, animal or human, or Asura. She was very tired and slept at once.

Satya-vatī awoke to a chilly dawn. She quickly roused the fire back to life. As the flames swelled, she took a small pan from her bag and roasted forest nuts over the fire, earnestly inviting Viṣṇu to enter the fire, enjoy the nuts, and allow her to then eat them as his gift. Viṣṇu famously accepted his devotee's offering, but then returned it to his devotee in a sanctified state that raised the devotee's consciousness.

Again, Satya felt the unseen Lord in the fire. When her offering was complete, she tasted his mercy in her abstemious breakfast of roasted nuts and cool river water.

As she prepared to journey down the river, she contemplated the apparent absurdity of her situation. Her sudden, brief encounter with Sau-nandya, a handsome, chivalrous, but clearly non-royal, stranger drove home that absurdity. Parā-śara promised her she would marry a king whom she could love, and who, she reasoned, could help her family in their struggle against the Asuras. But even Sau-nandya, a commoner, had assumed her to be as common, or probably more common, than himself. How a proper prince or king could possibly propose to a country girl wandering aimlessly down the Yamunā, entirely eluded her imagination. Yet, for her son's safety, and her own, she must continue to present herself to the world as just such a girl. If common men were attracted to her beauty, that made things worse. She would constantly have to fend them off, and deal with their belief that she thought too highly of herself.

When she added to these wretched thoughts her rational fear for her brothers and their children, before the rising Asura power, she could not fight off the misery that seized her mind and heart. Jarā-sandha grew steadily stronger, and Śan-tanu protected only his own growing domain and nothing more.

And all that my father worked so hard for may now be ruined, she thought. Only her faith in Parā-śara's words gave her strength to go on.

She brooded her way down the river, no happier than she was in the fishing village. But she was determined to seek her fortune. As the sun went low, she stopped to camp at a riverside clearing not very different from the one she left that morning.

The next morning, unable to rouse her spirits, she again decided that a change of scenery might distract her. She bowed to goddess Yamunā, beseeched her help, and continued her journey, seeking happiness around every bend.

After several days, and a few stops to rest and gather forest fare to eat, she guided her boat into a wide inlet, bordered by soft sand and coconut trees. She decided to return to the spiritual practice she had learned in the Final Forest, and sat down on the sand to meditate.

But the same depressing thoughts disturbed her meditation. She could bear the grief and loneliness no longer. Overwhelmed, she wept and cried out uncontrollably, her tears falling on the sand.

Then, she sensed with alarm that someone was nearby. She looked up and saw Sau-nandya standing at a distance, watching her intently.

CHAPTER 20

"Forgive my intrusion," he said softly, "but I happened upon you, and I could not leave you in this state. Is there anything I can do to help?"

Too exhausted and forlorn to be embarrassed, she wiped her eyes and said in a choked voice, "You again? Are you following me?"

"I'm afraid it is me again. But I swear I'm not following you. In fact, assuming you were traveling downstream, my footprints on the river trail prove that I came from the opposite direction."

Satya-vatī could not help smiling at this proffered evidence.

"I believe you," she said. "I won't check your footprints."

He smiled. "May I tell you something?"

"Yes, say whatever you like."

"Thank you. I assure you that I was earnestly trying to avoid you, though only because you seem to find my company unpleasant. But now, seeing you unhappy, I will be very sorry if I cannot help you in some way. I say that with deep respect for an honorable lady. I speak as a soul who cares about other souls, if I may borrow your words."

"Thank you," she said. "I trust your kind intention. I apologize if I offended you in any way when we first met."

"Truly, you made no offense. I respected you all the more for the strict propriety of your conduct."

She thanked him for this compliment with a short bow.

"I am a soldier," he said, "and I have been trained to help those in distress. So, both instinct and training incline me to help you, if I can. I have no other intention, on my honor."

He spoke these words so earnestly that Satya believed him, and her attitude softened into equally sincere cordiality. "When we last met, you introduced yourself as Sau-nandya. I am Satya-vatī. I grew up in a village several hours up the sacred Yamunā." She could not reveal to this stranger her birth family, nor would she falsely state that she was a fisherman's daughter. If only she was free to tell the truth. She had better change the subject. And she did want to know more about this chivalrous soldier.

"Forgive my curiosity," she said. "I have no wish to invade your privacy. But if you are a soldier, why are you here, so far from any king's army?"

"That is a reasonable question. May I sit?"

"Yes, of course."

He bowed his head, and sat at a respectful distance. With a sigh, he began. "I suffered a great disappointment in my life, and I had the opportunity to get away for some time from a place that constantly reminded me of my loss."

Satya saw the pain in the soldier's eyes as he spoke these words. His manner made clear that he would not welcome questions on the exact nature of his loss.

"If I may ask," he said, "why were you so sad? Can I help in any way?"

"Thank you. But I don't think either of us can solve my problem." She would not be more open or explicit than him. After he was so vague about his own grief, she gave a vague reply to his question.

"I too have been disappointed," she said, "though I am grateful for my blessings."

"Of course. And I hope that even in my grief, I too am grateful for my blessings."

"And we must not simply think of our own problems," Satya said. "The world too has problems and disappointments."

"It certainly does," he said. Seeing his pleasure in her company, Satya resolved at once not to say or do anything that might encourage him to aspire to her. She was dressed in a common way, but her duty and destiny was to marry royalty. He was a regular soldier, however handsome and well spoken. So she took the conversation in another direction, away from their personal lives. "I'm sad because the world is in danger, yet mighty kings care more about their own status and power than about the innocent people they are sworn to serve."

"You concern yourself with these matters?" he asked.

"Why should I not?"

"No reason, it is certainly your right."

"Thank you. The state of the world does concern me. Everyone knows how well the late King Vasu protected this Earth."

"Yes," Sau-nandya said, "the world certainly knows that King Vasu was a great man, a great king, indeed, an emperor."

"Yes, and he acted unselfishly. That is my point."

"Do you feel that leaders today are selfish in comparison?"

"I think some of them are selfish, since you ask."

"Do you have any particular kings in mind?"

"I don't know you, Sau-nandya, and so perhaps I should not speak freely on this subject. I might offend your monarch, or one whom you revere."

"Please don't worry about that. Tell me what you think. I will listen carefully, and tell you honestly if my view varies from yours. In my country, we have a long tradition of speaking freely, even about kings. We do not hesitate to praise or criticize a king as we see fit. And I would very much like to hear your view. You will not offend me by stating your opinion."

Satya-vatī smiled. "In that case, my honest opinion is that the Kuru lord Śan-tanu is far too proud. Indeed, he is dangerously proud."

"Interesting. Perhaps he is," Sau-nandya said. "But why do you say that?"

"I heard that King Vasu's sons, all noble kings, seek Śan-tanu's friendship, so that together they can protect our world from, well, all possible attacks. You yourself spoke of Asuras taking birth as beasts, and you must know those beasts are attacking innocent sages. Those who govern and protect us must be prepared for any type of threats. But Śan-tanu thinks himself too good for the Cedi lords. Lord Indra himself favored our King Vasu. And why would Indra personally come to this world and empower the great Vasu, if there was not a very serious threat to our planet?"

Sau-nandya nodded. "You ask a most cogent question. Why indeed would Indra himself come to this small world, and give such power to King Vasu, were there not a serious problem? Please go on."

Satya-vatī thanked him and said, "Precisely. Vasu protected the world when Śan-tanu was a mere child. Yet Śan-tanu, with no crystal aircraft, no similar mandate from Indra, now thinks that he can protect the world alone. He seems to underestimate the possible dangers."

"Perhaps he does," Sau-nandya said, deep in thought.

"Yes, and in doing so, he may be endangering the world. And all this, apparently, for his pride. Perhaps he resents that Indra shifted the traditional leadership of Hastinā-pura to Cedi. Śan-tanu forgets that Vasu himself was a Kuru, and that his family also has Kuru blood, and is most pious and trustworthy."

"I'm sure Śan-tanu reveres Vasu. But he may have less confidence in Vasu's sons. I mean no offense. I am simply speculating on what the Kuru king might think. After all, after inheriting the Kuru nation from his father, Śan-tanu basically had to rebuild the celebrated Kuru army. King Pratīpa saw no danger and planned for none. It was Śan-tanu who clearly saw how vulnerable his nation actually was. And in that state, he was naturally wary of other great world powers."

Concealing her anger at this argument, Satya-vatī said, "I respect Śan-tanu's need to rebuild the Kuru force. And I respect his caution while doing so. But that should have made him more, not less, eager for a Cedi alliance. Whatever the relative power of Vasu's sons, no one has ever doubted their character as noble kings. How can their word be doubted? Or their motives? They risked their lives, fighting by their father's side, against the Asuras."

Sau-nandya listened ever more intently. "Please go on," he said.

"I have only this to add. In mistrusting their intentions and their character, Śan-tanu offends Vasu's faithful sons. I have heard that all five would welcome an alliance with Śan-tanu. But he rebuffs them, as if their overtures were false, self-interested, or of no value."

"How do you know all this?" Sau-nandya asked.

Satya-vatī colored and said, "I have an acquaintance, a friend, who intimately serves the royal family. I gave that person my word that I would not reveal their identity."

"Of course. I honor your integrity. Indeed, all that you say is most interesting."

Satya quickly added, "I mean no offense to the Kuru lord. I truly wish him well, but I must speak the truth as I see it."

Sau-nandya gazed at Satya-vatī. "I find your view most interesting. Indeed, your honesty is refreshing. I know you speak what you truly believe. And your beliefs are rational. Śan-tanu has astute ministers, but they are Kurus to the core. He may not ever hear opinions like yours."

"Thank you for listening," Satya-vatī said. "I repeat that I mean no offense to Śan-tanu. But his behavior seems hard to bear."

Sau-nandya smiled. "Given your view of the geo-political situation, I can see why you hold the Kuru king in such low esteem."

"Be honest. Do you consider my view biased or partial?"

Sau-nandya pressed his lips together, as if choosing his words with care. "I am wondering whether some personal motive might influence Śan-tanu and prevent him from thinking clearly on these matters. It does seem likely that Śan-tanu lamented, even resented, the transfer of power from Hastinā-pura to Cedi. Yet I'm sure he understood the logic of Indra's decision. Now that I've heard you, I wonder if Śan-tanu's policies are being driven by that resentment, rather than purely strategic calculations."

Satya-vatī said, "Thank you for hearing me. Perhaps Śan-tanu has more noble motives, but really, what could they possibly be?"

Sau-nandya smiled. "If I am to defend Śan-tanu's motives, I will surely disappoint you."

"Really?"

"Yes. After hearing from you, I fear that I do not know exactly what motivates that man. Few of us perfectly understand our deepest motives. This may be true of Śan-tanu. A king's life is not always conducive to the humility necessary for true self-knowledge. How can I defend a man who may not know himself?"

"Very true," Satya said. Sau-nandya's reasoning pleased her. She admired much about him. If only he were royalty, she might envision a life with him. But she could not indulge in dangerous, impossible fantasies. She knew that social rank did not define the soul. But she also knew that souls living in this world must perform their duties, lest chaos reign.

Parā-śara promised she would marry, with love, a powerful noble who could protect her from Asuras and facilitate her service to all the Avatāras. A strategic alliance, formed by marrying a man she loved, would make a crucial difference in defending Earth and the devoted warriors who would risk, and sacrifice, their lives to defend it. She would not trivialize their sacrifice by a purely self-serving union, in the name of romance.

Sau-nandya's social position did not prevent her from respecting him, admiring and befriending him in a proper, circumscribed way. Had their positions been different, she might have considered him as a possible partner in her life. But all that was impossible.

Anxious now to abandon their heavy discussion of Śan-tanu in favor of less depressing topics, she said, "Sau-nandya, I hope you are enjoying your tour of the Yamunā region."

He smiled, pleased at her interest in his affairs. "Yes, I am. I'd always heard that Yamunā is a kind goddess, and I've found it to be true. She is kind indeed."

"Oh yes, Yamunā is most kind to those who seek her."

"Satya-vatī, I suspect that you are equally kind."

"Please, sir, do not compare me to Yamunā. I am but her humble servant."

"Of course," Sau-nandya said. "But has no one ever told you how much you resemble a goddess?"

Satya-vatī stood up at once. "Excuse me, sir, but there cannot be such talk between us." Many had compared her beauty to that of a goddess, but her heart was opening to this stranger, and that was dangerous. Seeing that her words disturbed him, she said, "I hope I didn't speak to you unkindly."

He sighed. "No, you did your duty and I thank you for it."

"What do you mean?"

"I fear I was growing too fond of you. I will not presume that you felt that way toward me." Actually, she did. He continued, "And since we can never marry, it is best that we separate."

"Yes, you are right," she said with a sigh of her own, "but how did you discover that we cannot marry?"

"I discovered it as soon as I saw you. I don't mean that I found any fault in you, for indeed, I did not. But I realized that society would not look kindly on our union, due to our very different situations in life."

"You refer to our respective social positions?" she asked.

"Yes, I do."

She nodded. How could he have discovered her identity? His discovery worried her, for other, less friendly persons might also know. Still, she could not help but be gratified that this attractive gentleman knew that she was royalty. "You are right," she said, "and as we know, Law and custom have their reasons, which the impulsive and the overly romantic cannot grasp."

"Precisely," he said. "The different social orders have different duties, different natures."

"Yes. For example," here she spoke from experience, "an ordinary girl may fall in love with a young sage, but their natures would be so different that a union between them must be problematic, regardless of any mutual attachment."

"Yes, exactly. So you do see the problem," he said. "Indeed, it is best to respect that Dharma which enjoins unions based on deeper nature, and not surface infatuation. Doubt does arise in cases where one feels that, against external custom, another person truly shares one's deeper nature." He sighed. "But in dangerous times like these, caution must define our duty. Anyway, I'm glad you also see that."

"Yes, of course I do," she replied, grasping his deeper meaning.

"Yes, of course. So, you were right. It is best that I not praise you as I did. And sadly, the only way I can avoid praising you is to say goodbye. I must do that now. Satya-vatī, with all my heart, I pray I did not offend you in any way, nor create a false expectation."

"Indeed, you did not," she said, missing him already, but seeing the need to separate.

"Then let us part as well-wishers and friends."

"Yes," she said sadly, "we will always be...well-wishers and friends."

They bowed to each other. He turned to leave and began walking toward his horse waiting at a distance. Suddenly, he turned and said, "I'm sorry, but before I go, I must ask you one question, for my own understanding."

"Please, ask," she said, bracing herself. What would he ask?

"Kindly tell me," he said, "how did you see through my disguise?"

"Your disguise?" At once she saw the painful truth. In stating the imprudence of a match between them, Sau-nandya was not speaking of his inferiority. He was speaking of hers.

"I don't understand," she said. "You told me you are a soldier. Are you not a soldier?"

"I am in fact a soldier," he said, walking back toward her. "But I...let us say that I concealed my rank."

This mortified her. He considered her so low that even a military officer could not marry her. Crestfallen, she asked, "So, what is your rank? Are you an officer in some king's army?"

He lowered his head. "No, not an officer. I am a king. I lead my army. I am truly sorry that I did not reveal this sooner."

Startled, fearing for his mental health, she said, "I don't understand. I know all the kings of this world by name and reputation, and there is no King or Prince Sau-nandya in this world."

"I did not lie to you," he said, looking quite embarrassed. "My mother's name is Su-nandā..."

"Of course, so one of your names is Sau-nandya, son of Su-nandā. May I then presume that the world knows you by a different name?"

"Yes, it does. The world knows me as Śan-tanu, king of the Kurus."

CHAPTER 21

So shocking was this revelation that Sau-nandya was the Kuru lord Śan-tanu, that Satya-vatī could hardly control the tempest of emotions that flooded her mind. The heaviest were the following.

Satya was mortified to have heavily criticized the Kuru monarch to his face, without knowing who he was.

She was outraged that he misled her into thinking he was someone else. He had befriended her on false pretenses.

She was confused. Having found him handsome, intelligent, and kind, she now learned that, as a king, he was eligible to marry her.

Śan-tanu had the power to help solve the world's problems, if he would cooperate with Cedi. She could not be selfish and think only of herself.

Śan-tanu looked equally mortified, which could only mean that he cared very much about her feelings. He had no reason to be outraged or shocked, since he could not imagine her real identity.

Too disturbed to talk, too embarrassed to stay there, Satya-vatī quickly put on her sandals and began walking on a sandy beach that bordered the wide inlet. In her agitated state, she did not fasten her sandals well, and tripped awkwardly along the trail. Śan-tanu caught up with her. She thought it best to stop and speak with him.

But neither spoke. After a mutually awful few minutes of silence, during which each tried hard to understand their own feelings, and that of the other, Satya-vatī faced him directly and said, "You didn't tell me when we met that you are Śan-tanu. I didn't know."

"Forgive me," he said, looking down. "I did not lie to you, but I did deceive you. I beg your forgiveness."

Without replying, she arranged her sandals, and walked slowly along the path, glancing back at him to indicate that he had her permission to walk with her. He understood and followed. How could she blame him, when she had not revealed her own identity?

She stopped. They faced each other. "I hope," he said, "I'm not making things worse, but I did have reasons to conceal my identity."

"Kindly reveal them," she said, inviting him to walk alongside her. She was too emotionally spent to quarrel. He thanked her, and as they walked along the water, he began his defense in a calm, gentle voice.

"First, as I told you before, I suffered a great disappointment, and I was desperate to escape the public sphere, to spend time in a peaceful place where I could remain incognito, and recover my spirit. So, once outside my realm, I traveled as Sau-nandya. I told you exactly what I told everyone. I never imagined I would see you again. So, when we first met, I saw much good, and no harm, in concealing my identity."

As bright, tropical birds flew past them, vanishing into the forest, Satya nodded and said, "So far, your story is reasonable, and I accept it. But did you allude to other considerations?"

"Yes, I did. When we met, I could hardly expect a simply dressed country maiden, or man, to have a mature command of geo-political issues. When you began to voice strong opinions about me, I wanted to hear your uncensored views about me, and world affairs in general. This was not mere curiosity. I had never heard such an able defense of the Cedi perspective. I have received overtures from Cedi kings, but the language was diplomatic and cautious. You were neither."

Satya could not help smiling at this accurate description. As cool river breezes refreshed them, she found herself enjoying her talk with the Kuru king. "All things considered," she said, "I might have done the same." In fact, she had done exactly what he did, and was still doing it — concealing her identity. It now struck her as absurd to blame him for an act that she also performed, and indeed continued to perpetuate long after he revealed himself.

As they walked along, she caught his eyes and smiled in a way that brought instant reciprocation from Śan-tanu.

"I imagine," she said in a convivial tone, "that you are surrounded by those who tend to praise and obey you."

"Yes, I am," he said, reciprocating her relaxed, friendly tone. "I'm sure you know how dangerous that can be. That's why I was so eager to hear from you what you truly think, unsoftened by the demands of diplomacy and decorum."

Satya laughed. "Another fair point. I am disarmed. But I do have a question."

His smile encouraged her to ask it. But before she could, loud, anguished cries broke the still air. They both looked down the beach, and saw a small crowd of people shouting for help. Śan-tanu and Satya-vatī ran toward them.

They found a small group of workers who lived by scaling the tall, thin trees and tossing coconuts down to their companions. A boy had slipped from high up, and plunged onto a stone at the tree's base. His frantic friends failed to stop the blood that poured from the unconscious boy's head wound.

Śan-tanu was a large, strongly built man, and as he ran swiftly up to the workers, those not directly attending the injured boy stepped aside in deference. Śan-tanu rushed to the boy, fell to his knees, and placed his hands directly on the wound, shielding it from view.

Śan-tanu closed his eyes, as if in meditation. When he lifted up his hands, covered in the boy's blood, the wound had vanished! The boy opened his eyes, looked around, and asked what had happened. With joyous shouts, his friends rushed to him. He was just as before, and soon stood up.

Meanwhile, Śan-tanu walked to the river and Satya-vatī watched him clean his hands in the sacred water. As she walked toward him, all the workers rushed past her, and showered praise and thanks on Śan-tanu, who seemed embarrassed by the attention. He insisted that Viṣṇu had saved their friend and urged them to take more care when climbing trees. The workers vowed they would. In heartfelt words, they thanked Śan-tanu again and again.

As they bowed to him, he bowed to them and bid them farewell. As they continued to cheer him, he walked straight to Satya-vatī and asked if they could leave. She agreed. As they walked back to their camp, Satya said, "Would you rather I not ask you about what I just saw?"

He stopped and said, "I guess it was a bit unusual."

"Oh yes!" Satya said. She looked quizzically at Śan-tanu and said, "Your Majesty, there is something I wanted to ask you, but I was too shy to do so."

"Really? I didn't find you exactly shy with me."

"I have certainly not been generally shy with you, but on one topic I did hesitate to speak. I will do so now."

"By all means," he said.

She thanked him and, gathering her courage, began. "Clearly, you have healing power in your hands. I have witnessed it."

"Yes, that is true."

"So, before we met, when I fell from your horse, I must have been seriously injured. And you healed me. Is that right?"

He looked down. "Yes, it is."

"Imagine that," she said. "I'd heard that the Kuru lord heals with his hands, but I assumed it was an exaggerated tale. I thought you had done it, but I was embarrassed to speak of it, since I didn't know you. But now I am comfortable to speak of it."

He laughed. "Perhaps you weren't hurt as badly as you thought."

"I think I was," she said, "and let me now thank you for my present good health."

Śan-tanu bowed and smiled. She said, "Where did you get this healing power?"

"It's simply a gift I received from the Devas when I came to this world in their service."

At that moment, Satya wanted to give him a big hug for saving that boy, and herself. But they still did not know each other well enough for that. Instead, they walked along in silence, till Satya felt she could do him a favor by bringing up a different topic. "You told me that you left the north and traveled here to escape an unhappy situation. I do not want to invade your privacy, but...what happened? I ask because I really want to understand you."

"I'm flattered that you wish to understand me," Śan-tanu said. "But I hesitate to burden you with my troubles."

"Please believe me," she said. "I truly wish to hear your story, if you feel you can share it. You see, I do care about you — even if you are Śan-tanu." She spoke these last words in a tone of mock horror, and he laughed heartily. Satya was pleased that he did not resent her past criticism. They were becoming close friends.

She added, "Whatever the future may hold for us, let us be open with each other. Let us be good friends."

"Yes! We shall be true friends. I will tell you my story, but promise me you will also tell yours."

She didn't expect this. No clever evasion came to her mind. "Yes," she said, concealing her great anxiety. "I promise."

Her words pleased Śan-tanu. "Let me just consider for a moment," he said, "how to begin my story." As he gathered his thoughts, they continued walking along the wide inlet. Birdsong filled the air. The tireless river sent soft waves lapping at the shore.

In asking about his life, Satya-vatī had a hidden motive — to see whether she could love him, and whether he could really love her. His behavior toward his first wife, the reason for her departure, and his response to it, would all reveal vital information about his character. Only then could Satya decide whether to employ the power she felt she possessed to fully win his love. Not knowing her royal blood, he believed they could never marry. Just as he had studied her before revealing his true identity, so now she would study him before he learned she was an emperor's daughter, most qualified to be his wife. But in securing his agreement to tell his story, she had committed to telling hers. How would she do it?

"Ready?" he asked.

Satya forced a smile. "I am eager to hear your story. You may depend on my confidentiality."

"It is a relief," he said, "to finally unburden myself to a friend, far removed from the political intrigue of a king's court."

He began his tale. "I met goddess Gaṅgā in my previous life in the Deva world. We felt an immediate attraction. Soon after, I learned that I must take birth again on Earth to help defeat an imminent Asura invasion. I'm sure you will keep this information confidential."

"Of course."

Śan-tanu thanked her and continued. "When the time came for me to return to Earth, Gaṅgā and I were in love. She insisted on coming with me. I warned her that as a goddess, she might not be happy here. But her mind was made up, and of course I was thrilled that she was coming."

"Did Gaṅgā actually take birth from a human couple?"

"No. That was too much for her. She waited in Deva-loka until I was grown and ready to marry. Then she simply rose out of her own waters and we were reunited."

"That is very romantic," Satya-vatī said, listening closely. "Please go on."

"We had a happy life together. We begot an excellent son, Deva-vrata. I thought our life would go on in that way. But, after some time, Gaṅgā wearied of life on Earth. Indeed, she found it unbearable. And so reluctantly, she returned to Deva-loka."

"I see that it's difficult for you to talk about it. I'm sorry."

"Please don't be sorry. Somehow, since meeting you, for the first time I don't feel the pain."

Satya colored. She must see whether Śan-tanu could truly love another woman, and this new information was invaluable. Clearly, she was special to him. But whether that special regard could develop into the full love of a devoted husband must be seen. Until she was sure that it could, she would not reveal her identity, nor encourage him in his affection for her.

At her request, he continued. "I remember well the day Gaṅgā left. I paced the palace frantically, struggling to overcome the pain in my heart. The sun had risen over the capital. She would be leaving soon. I knew that. But I had to make one last appeal. I walked to her private quarters, hardly feeling the floor beneath me. I pushed through the jeweled curtains to her antechamber. A lady-in-waiting appeared and bowed."

Śan-tanu stopped, lost in sad memories. Satya-vatī waited patiently. He continued. "I told the attendant I wished to see the queen. She looked at me with a face so miserable, it cruelly confirmed the futility of my attempt. Gaṅgā appeared, begged my forgiveness, thanked me for all I had done, spoke kind words, bid me farewell, and vanished as the celestials do. She took our son, promising to return him after the Devas had trained him."

"I can imagine how painful that was," Satya said, remembering the loss of her own son, and Parā-śara.

Śan-tanu bowed. "Thank you. I must be boring you with these stories. Everyone has their troubles."

"No, not at all," she exclaimed. "Please go on. What did you do then?"

"At first, I vowed not to suffer from her absence. If she would not stay for my sake, I would not suffer for hers. She would not rob me of my joy in life. I would encounter pleasure or pain from my own deeds and decisions, not hers. But my vow proved futile. I did suffer very much. And worse, Gaṅgā's sacred waters flow within view of my palace. I could not forget her, and that made my life unbearable. I had to get away from Hastinā-pura. Everything there reminded me of her."

Satya-vatī nodded, and remained silent. She wondered if Śan-tanu could ever really love another woman, after losing a goddess. With a compassionate glance, she encouraged him to continue. He did.

"Well, I was deeply depressed, defeated, hopeless. Everyone urged me to stay — advisors and generals, all the citizens — but when they saw my grief, they understood."

"Of course, they care about you."

"Yes, they do. And I am most grateful. But I had to get away. I assured them I would return soon, and were there any real emergency, I would come at once. But I craved peace and solitude. I had to get far away. And I know you understand that a Kuru king cannot just wander through other people's kingdoms. Were I detected, it would violate political protocol and create a commotion. So, I adopted my maternal name, dressed as a common man, and set out to see the world, to forget."

Satya's heart filled with compassion. "That is fully understandable. Of course you had to travel incognito."

"And I could not travel along the Gaṅgā, for obvious reasons."

"Yes, that is equally clear. But why did you come to this region? The mighty Himālayas are not far from your capital, and there you would have found peace, beauty, and solitude."

"Yes, but Gaṅgā and I had often vacationed in the great mountains, so it was not a safe place to recover from her loss. I went south. I was curious to see the new kingdom of Matsya."

Satya-vatī concealed her amazement. "Did you meet King Matsya there?"

"No, I didn't. I didn't want to risk detection."

"Of course." Satya-vatī tried to act calm. "And how did you find the new kingdom?"

Śan-tanu smiled. "I liked it very much. The city is lovely, built of red sandstone. Nature there is quite beautiful, and the people were all kind. The young king is quite popular. He treats his people well. Perhaps I'll meet him someday."

"Yes, perhaps you will." To herself, Satya said, If you marry me, you will meet him sooner than you expect.

"So," she said with forced tranquility, "how did you get from there to here?"

Śan-tanu smiled. "I didn't want to go west into the great desert or east into Śūra-sena. The royalty knows me there. I was not ready to return north. I had no choice but to continue south. I decided to go on pilgrimage to Yamunā's purifying waters. I hoped the goddess would relieve my suffering."

"Oh yes!" Satya cried. "Yamunā is most kind. She has always comforted me through my travails. Did you find relief?"

"Yes, I did. I even believe that goddess Yamunā made a most unexpected, but most welcome arrangement. And now I am happy."

Satya-vatī knew well that he was speaking of her, but she chose not to respond or react to his words. Not yet. Instead, she said, "I think I know why you traveled to Yamunā in this specific area."

Śan-tanu smiled. "Really? You think you know?"

"Yes, but I do not wish to interrupt you."

"Not at all! Please tell me. I'm curious."

Satya smiled playfully. "Of course, I merely conjecture. However, it seems quite simple. When you left the land of Matsya, you wished to visit Yamunā, but you could not take the shortest route to the East, because then you would pass through Śūra-sena, which you wanted to avoid. Nor could you take a circuitous route through Pañcāla, since you must be well known there as well. Pañcāla borders the Kuru land. Thus, you traveled southeast into Cedi, where you are far less known. And that is how you came to this area and met me. Am I right?"

Śan-tanu laughed. "You are very clever, Satya-vatī. Indeed, you are unlike anyone I've ever known — audacious and reserved, innocent and shrewd. Forgive me. I know you don't like to be praised."

"That is true." She smiled.

"And now, it is your turn."

"My turn?"

"Yes, of course," he said. "You must tell me about your life, and what you are doing all alone in this forest."

"Yes, I did promise." Satya had no escape.

CHAPTER 22

How much could she reveal? If she could love him, she must explain her royal birth, so that marriage was possible. If she could not love him, she would explain only her life as a fishing girl. Indeed, her low background would quickly banish any notion of marriage from his mind.

It took her but a moment to decide. She could love him. Maybe she already did. A voice in her heart whispered that by her influence, he would become fully the king he should be. His account of Gaṅgā's departure satisfied her. It perfectly matched all she had heard. And if true, Śan-tanu was blameless.

But with all that, she would only marry him if he accepted her brothers as family. He would thus put the world's good, and her own, above any misguided manly pride. She could only broach this topic when he knew her to be high royalty, eligible to be his bride. Parā-śara had promised her a loving, royal marriage. Hesitation and doubt now vanished. She would reveal herself, and see Śan-tanu's reaction.

Satya-vatī took a deep breath and said, "I will now tell you about my life, but first I will say this. I believe you care about me as much as I care about you. But you must marry royalty. That is your conflict. Is it not?"

He sighed in resignation. "Yes, it is, since you state it so openly. But how does this preface the story of your life?"

"Because I felt the same conflict about you that you feel about me."

Śan-tanu stared at her. "What do you mean? What conflict did you feel?"

"You, Śan-tanu, presented yourself as a good but ordinary man, not as royalty. Therefore, though I liked you very much, I concluded that I could not marry you."

Śan-tanu's eyes opened wide. "Do you mean that you are royalty?"

"Yes, I am royalty. The world does not know my real identity."

Too astonished to be calm, and still staring, Śan-tanu cried, "Satya-vatī, who are you?"

"I will tell you, but only if you vow upon your honor that you will never reveal my secret, unless we marry."

"You have my word as Kuru king that if I do not marry you, I will never reveal your secret. To anyone."

Satya-vatī nodded. "I trust you. No Kuru king would ever break his vow. Śan-tanu, as you were born of the celebrated and saintly King Pratīpa and his revered wife, Queen Su-nandā, so I was born to one praised by all as the king of kings. My father is King Vasu, and my mother is his illustrious wife, Queen Girikā."

Amazed beyond speech, Śan-tanu gazed at Satya-vatī as if tracing out the lines of her exalted birth in her exquisite face. At last, he said, "The world does not know that great Vasu had a daughter. How did you come to live in a remote village as a simple maiden, you who are the most noble princess on Earth? Forgive me for asking. Such a noble family must have their reasons. But you know why I must ask."

"I do. It is shocking, perhaps unbelievable, that a noble family would conceal their only daughter and send her away to live a poor life. I see no impropriety in your question. I myself was no less shocked when I first learned my real identity. But it is true. I am the twin sister of King Matsya, through whose kingdom you recently passed. If you meet him, you will see our striking resemblance."

Śan-tanu looked upon her as upon a great wonder. "Forgive me, but I cannot rest until I know your story. You promised to tell me."

"I will tell you at once why I was sent away, and given a false identity, by the order of Indra himself."

Śan-tanu raised his eyebrows. "Indra himself. I beg you, explain."

Satya saw the admiration in Śan-tanu's expression. Gazing fearlessly into his eyes, she explained every pertinent fact related to her extraordinary life, including her absolute need to conceal her identity.

Śan-tanu listened to every syllable in a state of wonder. He saw his heart fully opening to her as she spoke.

Only on one point, for a higher purpose, did she intentionally mislead the Kuru king, when she said, "Lord Indra came to my parents and told them that invading Asuras had learned that I was destined to unite with a powerful soul, and that this union would pose a major obstacle to their invasion."

Satya-vatī knew Śan-tanu would assume that the powerful soul foretold by Indra was Śan-tanu himself, not Parā-śara. Factually, a union with Śan-tanu would unite the Kurus and Cedis, thus dealing a major blow to the Asuras.

She regretted having to use such artifice, but it was necessary, and she did not dwell on it. She could not fail in her duty to help save Earth. Her union with Śan-tanu, which must unite Kurus with Cedis, was essential. And, for the first time in her life, Satya-vatı was truly in love. Over two years had passed since she first met Parā-śara. She now saw clearly that her attachment to him had been a combination of deep reverence and youthful infatuation. But her attachment to Śan-tanu was the natural love of a woman for a worthy man.

Seeing Śan-tanu still astonished, Satya said, "You may ask any of my brothers to confirm my words."

Śan-tanu shook his head. "I would never dishonor you by seeking their confirmation. Indeed, I see from your bold spirit and noble mien that you were born of high royal blood. And we are both from the same noble dynasty. Your father was a Kuru, though he ruled Cedi."

Satya-vatī happily agreed.

Śan-tanu paused here. "Satya-vatī, I have one doubt that I pray you will remove. May I present it?"

"Of course," she said, anxiously wondering what it was.

"My doubt is this: your father, the great Vasu, whom we all revere, sent you away because he feared he could not protect you. If the danger is still so great, how will I protect you, once your identity is revealed? I do not fear the Asuras in battle. I myself came to Earth from the Deva realm. But I am not stronger than your revered father, yet he did not reveal your identity. You know my citizens will only accept our marriage if your royal identity is known. Satya-vatī, this is my quandary. I can never put you in danger. Will you be safe with me, once you reveal yourself to the world?"

Satya-vatī smiled. "I honor your concern. But I will be safe under your protection. At the time of my birth, we knew much less about the Asuras than we do now. Even Indra was uncertain. My loving parents chose not to risk my life. My father then killed many Asuras, making the world safer. By then, he feared that were my identity revealed, he would have to explain to the world why he sent me away."

Śan-tanu nodded. "And, since few know of the Asura invasion, people would panic, and the Asuras would target you."

"Precisely. Thus, my father could not reveal the truth. I suffered and doubted when I learned the truth, but I am now convinced that my parents acted out of love for me, and dedication to the world. But times have changed."

"Yes, they have."

"And the celebrated sage Parā-śara personally told me that I was destined to marry a great king who would be able to protect me. He said I could then reveal my true identity."

Śan-tanu exclaimed, "You spoke personally to Parā-śara?"

"Yes, I did. He was kind to me. He understood my situation."

"So, you are convinced that you would be safe with me?"

"Yes, I am confident of your protection. Also, if we marry, the mighty Kurus will form a natural alliance with my five brothers, the brave sons of Vasu. Śan-tanu, you must see that I, and the world, will be safer with a Kuru-Cedi alliance. And you must do me the honor of believing that if I married you merely to form an alliance, I would tell you so at once. But I could never marry you if I did not love you."

"And do you love me?"

Satya-vatī looked down. "Yes. I do. But tell me your heart. Do you love me enough—do you love the world enough—to accept my brothers as your brothers? Will you form an alliance with us? No matter how much I love you, I can only give my hand to one who loves those whom I love, one who cares about the world as much as I do. You alone can protect the Kuru realm, and neighboring states. But alone, you cannot protect the entire world. You are a great king and warrior, but you will be even stronger if you fight alongside my noble brothers."

Śan-tanu smiled. "Yes, I do love you enough to do all that you ask. I will do it gladly. But, dear Satya, if there is anything else you must tell me, say it now."

She then told him about her nephew Jarā-sandha, pointing out that this mighty Asura would become Śan-tanu's nephew as well.

"Oh, I knew about Jarā-sandha," he said.

"You did? But how?"

"Let us say that a Kuru king enjoys many channels of information that are not available to most rulers. Remember, in my last life I lived in Deva-loka. I have many friends there, including Indra. So, for now, your wicked nephew will become my wicked nephew. I know about the dreaded third generation. When it takes power, my son and our sons, allied with your nephews and other brave young kings, will have to contend with Jarā-sandha and other Asuras. For now, having Jarā-sandha as a nephew is not a problem. It's a sort of advantage. I will have easier access to him, and will more easily monitor his actions. So, is there any other issue we must discuss?"

"Yes, there is, dear king. Last, and most important, is this: you and I are eternal souls within our ephemeral bodies. I speak to you as one soul to another when I say that I will forever follow Viṣṇu. I've heard that you too are devoted to Viṣṇu. But I must hear it from you. Sages say that if Asuras grow too strong, Viṣṇu himself will come to this world. If Viṣṇu does come in our life, we must fight at his side. We cannot remain neutral."

A broad smile spread across Śan-tanu's face. Satya thought he had never looked so handsome. "If you could see within my heart," he said, "you would see Viṣṇu dwelling there. Satya-vatī, I will always fight with and for Viṣṇu."

"Now I fully believe you are the noble man that Parā-śara foretold would enter my life."

"With all my heart," he said, "I pray I am that man. But there is something I must tell you. Listen and tell me if you still want me."

"That sounds very serious," she said. "Tell me at once."

"It is this. You know I have a son, Deva-vrata."

"Of course. All the world knows that."

"Yes. Satya, by Law, Dharma, Deva-vrata will inherit the Kuru throne. Before I met you, I established him as Yuva-rāja, my heir apparent. Now, even I cannot legally deny him the throne, nor would I. Will you be happy with your stepson as Kuru heir? Our sons will be Kuru princes, and of course one day they will be kings, being so much younger than Deva-vrata."

Satya-vatī smiled and sighed with relief. "I'm glad your confession is only this. I very happily accept Deva-vrata as your heir."

Śan-tanu joyfully thanked her for that proof of her love for him. She then asked with some trepidation if Deva-vrata would accept her.

"Oh yes. Deva-vrata has the most generous heart in the world, and because he was separated from me almost at birth, and only returned four years ago, he is especially attached to me. The boy cannot bear to see me unhappy. He knows how I've suffered since his mother left, and he has often urged me to find a woman I can love. He is mature beyond his years, and devoted to my happiness. Seeing how happy you have made me, he will love you with all his heart. I only pray to be worthy of his devotion."

"I've heard that he is as handsome as his father, and that he has the power of a Deva."

Śan-tanu laughed. "As a proud father, I find him more handsome than me. And he certainly has extraordinary power. With the help of Deva-vrata, and a Kuru-Cedi alliance, the Asuras will be reluctant to attack."

"You are very fortunate to have such a son."

"Yes, but no more fortunate than to have found you. And someday, Satya, our sons will lend their strength to the cause."

Satya-vatī embraced him in her heart. She was now convinced that Viṣṇu had brought them together.

Śan-tanu stepped toward her. She did not step back. He took her hand. She did not withdraw it. He gazed into her eyes. "Dear Satya-vatī, now that we know each other's true identity, is there any reason why we should not unite?"

"No, there is not. But one thing worries me still."

Śan-tanu looked puzzled. "What can that be?"

"My dear Śan-tanu, I want to marry you. But how will you ever be satisfied with me, after living with a goddess? I fear you will always compare me to her, a comparison that must ever diminish me in your eyes. I am merely human, despite all your flattery."

"First," Śan-tanu replied, "you know as well as I that neither of us is ultimately celestial or human. We are both eternal souls, and it is your soul that attracts me. Satya-vatī, truly your heart and mind are as beautiful as your lovely face. Please believe that in my eyes, you can never suffer in comparison with any woman in the three worlds."

Satya smiled broadly. "If that be the case, then I see no reason why we should not unite in matrimony."

Śan-tanu beamed. "Let us go at once to Hastinā-pura."

"Yes, let us go."

By now, they had returned to the campsite where Śan-tanu's noble horse peacefully grazed. As they readied for the journey, Satya-vatī said, "Śan-tanu..."

"Yes?"

"If you don't mind, could we travel along the Yamunā? We will pass directly by the village where a loving fishing family raised me. They are good, simple people, and it would mean the world to them if we stopped there. It would make me happy if they met you and gave their blessings to our marriage. If you don't mind."

"I am delighted that I can so easily please you. Of course we will stop there. It is directly on the way. And I will personally thank those good souls who raised you."

"But I must warn you. They know nothing of my royal birth. It was kept secret from them for my safety."

"I understand. A wise decision. Give me but a moment, and I will bring our horse."

Satya-vatī thanked him, and sat alone on the bank of dear Yamunā. She knew that higher worlds existed. Indeed, her parents went to such a world. But as long as she remained on Earth, she could aspire to no greater happiness than to marry a man she loved, and thereby unite the Kurus with Cedi, and thus protect the Earth. Parā-śara's prophecy was indeed being fulfilled.

A rhythmic trotting roused her from her reverie. Śan-tanu, happier than she had ever seen him, approached on his proud steed.

CHAPTER 23

Śan-tanu dismounted and quickly packed Satya's things in his saddlebags. He tied her boat to the saddle. A little path ran along the river to a nearby village, and they had agreed to haul her boat there. Śan-tanu then would pay a boy to bring the boat back to Satya's village. Mounting his horse, he reached out, grasped Satya's hand, and easily lifted her onto the saddle behind him.

All was ready. "Hold on to me," the king said. With some shyness, for she had never held him, she wrapped her arms around his rock-solid waist. In her mind, Satya excitedly planned how they should tell her brothers the good news, the wonderful news!

They began their journey at a slow pace and were soon eagerly conversing. In a few minutes they dropped off her boat, and headed to a wider, faster road.

With the wind in her face, her hair trailing behind her, Satya-vatī wanted to laugh with joy. She asked Śan-tanu how she could best send the news to her brothers. He offered this plan. As soon as they were done in Kalpi, at the first town of greater size, he would send a Kuru agent anywhere she liked with the good news.

"You have Kuru agents in all the cities?" she asked.

"Of course!" he laughed, with a shrug of his shoulders. "It's what we have to do. I'm sure your brothers do the same."

"Yes, I'm sure they do," she said. She had never thought about it.

After an hour, they stopped by the river to briefly rest. Śan-tanu said, "Satya-vatī, when we first met, you spoke of a disappointment in your life. You never mentioned it again. Can you tell me about it?"

Satya smiled. "There's not much to tell. I met a young brāhmaṇa."

"And you fell in love with him?"

"To some extent. But he leads the quiet, meditative life of a sage. I am an emperor's daughter. I must be active."

He smiled with approval. Satya then made clear to him that her affections were not divided. He received her assurances happily.

At her inquiry, he spoke of his son, Deva-vrata, of whom the world heard so much. The boy was famously born to the goddess Gaṅgā, and grew up with her in the Deva world. No one in this world had yet discovered the limits of his strength. Satya-vatī listened eagerly, but sadly she could not reciprocate Śan-tanu's candor. She was forced to conceal the birth of her own son, Dvaipāyana, who also possessed unfathomable power.

She knew that Śan-tanu could never marry her if her connection with Parā-śara were known. She trusted that he would still accept her, but the unfair world would not. A scandal would arise, damaging the king's ability to rule. Most importantly, public knowledge of the still-young Avatāra might endanger him.

They rode for a while in silence, over bright green meadows and through flowering woods, keeping always near the river. Then, Satya-vatī asked if the Kuru kingdom was safe in his absence.

Śan-tanu smiled. "That is a most appropriate question from an emperor's daughter. Yes, the Kuru kingdom is in good hands. The army is strong. And everyone knows I am not so far away. I will be quickly informed of any suspicious troop movements on the part of humans or suspected Asuras. I send my agents everywhere. It is a duty I cannot avoid. For now, no one dares challenge Kuru power. I'll return soon, before I'm needed. And you will come with me. You will enter Hastinā-pura as my queen."

"Thank you," was all Satya could say, as wonder and gratitude filled her heart. Parā-śara had predicted her good fortune, but to enter the legendary imperial capital as the Kuru queen, and the queen of a king she loved, to play a key role in forging an alliance that could save Earth — all this surpassed by far what Satya-vatī had dared imagine possible when Parā-śara promised her future joy.

The fine horse trotted along, reaching a large village. "I long to say," the king said, "that you are as lovely as a Devī from the Deva realm. But I fear you will chastise me if I say it, as you once did."

Satya-vatī smiled. "You just said it. And I admonished you then for your compliment, because we did not know each other well."

He nodded. "And I respected you for admonishing me. It showed character. But now I can say it. And we have arrived at the village."

He slid off the horse, and lifted her down. They agreed that he would inquire about the fastest road to Kalpi, and she would purchase their lunch. With an arch smile, she said, "You will have to give me a few coins for that, if you can spare them." He laughed and complied.

Satya wandered through the village, conversing easily with the people. She spoke their language. This village was more prosperous than her own. A few fine homes on elevated land, with river views, revealed that affluent traders lived here.

Wherever she walked, people stared at her in wonder, for she did look as lovely as a goddess. She purchased their lunch and a cloth to wrap it. She heard a voice calling her. She turned and saw Śan-tanu approaching, leading two fine horses, his own and another.

"I bought this horse for you. You'll be more comfortable on our trip. It's a fine horse that belonged to the local mayor."

Delighted at this gift, Satya brought Śan-tanu to a grassy knoll on the riverbank and spread out their lunch on the large cloth. Breezes, blowing over Yamunā's cool waters, refreshed them. Chatting and laughing like old friends, they relished their lunch, and were soon mounted for their ride toward Satya's village. They left this village without anyone imagining their identity.

Now the great king and the emperor's daughter were free to gallop through the countryside. They rode joyfully through rich green meadows, and varicolored woodlands that were bright and fragrant with fruits and flowers. Satya had never been happier. As the wind rushed over her face and blew back her hair, she laughed with sheer joy.

After a while, they stopped to let their horses rest and drink from Yamunā's life-giving waters. They sat together on the grassy bank, watching the endless currents roll by. The river sparkled in the bright sun.

Śan-tanu bowed and smiled. "Well, I am eager to see the bucolic village where you grew up."

"I wish it had been bucolic, idyllic," she said. "But you will see soon enough." And without another word, she dove into the sacred Yamunā, popped her head up, and challenged him to race across the river.

He looked around, saw no one nearby, and unfastened his sword belt. Patting the horses, telling them to stay, he kicked off his shoes and dove into the water.

Satya laughed and took off for the far bank. He went after her with powerful arms, but she had grown up as much in water as on land.

He could not catch her, though he stayed close behind. Reaching the far bank, she turned and laughed as he approached. His laughter merged with hers.

They returned to the other shore floating on their backs, joking and bantering all the way. The hot tropical sun soon dried them and their clothes. They mounted their horses and rode happily along the river.

As Satya-vatī and Śan-tanu came ever closer to her village, Satya realized that these might be some of their most carefree moments together, without the constraints of palace pomp or formality. Once married, it would be hard to fully escape the duties, decorum, and protocol of Kuru royalty.

She sought to savor these moments as they splashed through crystalline streams, loped over meadows carpeted with wildflowers, and cantered through haunting woods. All along the way, no one recognized either of them — the emperor's daughter and the world's most powerful king.

As they approached her village, and the scenery grew increasingly familiar, and depressing, Satya found that guilt and foreboding filled her mind, not the joy of reunion and mutual appreciation that she first imagined. After much time away, she hoped her foster parents would appreciate her desire to share with them the joy of her engagement to a great king. This might be their last chance to see her for a long time, perhaps forever. They did not travel. Once established as Kuru Queen, Satya-vatī was not likely to return.

Recalling how her foster parents had always opposed her lofty ambitions, she now feared that all of Śan-tanu's fame and power might not satisfy such proud, plain people who had always sought to impose their plain ways on her. Even a glorious marriage to the Kuru king might not wash away their resentment of her for having rejected their home and their ways.

As they approached the village, every head turned. No one in the village had ever seen Satya on a horse. And a handsome man with a large, warrior's build had brought her! Feeling the stares, the royal pair dismounted and walked quietly toward the cottage of the fisher king, who stood in the doorway with his wife, staring at them in stark incredulity.

CHAPTER 24

The entire village surrounded the royal pair, trying as discreetly as possible — it was not very discreet — to overhear what was said. Seeing this, Dāśa-rāja, fisher king, invited his daughter and her tall friend into his cottage. There Satya at once made the introductions, explaining that the great Kuru king had been traveling incognito.

Dāśa-rāja and his wife stared at Śan-tanu with astonishment and incredulity. Their natural reverence for kings bent their bodies at the waist and lowered their heads, but their incredulity froze their bodies mid-bow, from where they looked up at him with questioning eyes.

Śan-tanu smiled and said, "Please don't trouble yourselves with formalities. I understand how strange it must seem to see me in this attire, and worse, accompanying your daughter before receiving your blessing. Forgive me for what appears to be an indiscretion; however, the circumstances of our meeting, and acquaintance, deprived us of the honor of seeking your prior blessings."

The fisher king's wife, hearing a voice and language that could only be that of a king, now completed her bow. Dāśa-rāja quickly followed her, making grand bows to the Kuru king that convinced Satya-vatī that it was a terrible mistake to bring Śan-tanu here.

When her foster father then began to explain that he was also a king of sorts, ruling the local fishing community, Satya was tempted to mount her horse and ride away. Seeing her discomfort, Dāśa-rāṇi intervened, inviting everyone to sit down to a hearty meal. Śan-tanu explained, with expressions of gratitude, that he had eaten recently, and so must decline her kind hospitality. After an awkward pause, Śan-tanu earnestly declared his intention to marry Satya-vatī, who anxiously studied her foster parents' reaction. As Śan-tanu spoke, Dāśa-rāja nodded politely, rocking back and forth in his seat. Her foster father was tight-lipped, grave, impenetrable. Satya knew that this mood portended some sort of trouble and she braced herself. When the Kuru king finished, the fisher king thanked him with a false humility that embarrassed Satya, and added, "O Kuru king, from my daughter's infancy, I knew that someday I would give her hand in marriage to a great man."

He turned to Satya-vatī. "Dear child, we raised you from infancy. We have no other child. You will break your mother's heart, and mine, if you marry without our blessings."

Her mother said, "Satya, we dedicated our lives to you. Promise us that you will take our blessings to marry."

Anxious to placate and silence her foster parents, Satya said, "Of course I will marry with your blessings. That's why we came here. So please, give us your blessings now."

The fisher king looked at his wife and they exchanged a knowing glance. Dāśa-rāja turned his gaze back to Satya-vatī. "Very good, my dear. Your name is Satya-vatī, the truthful one. Never did you break your promise, nor have you spoken a lie. And now that you are sworn to marry only with our blessings, we will give those blessings as soon as this mighty king agrees to a simple condition."

"Condition? What are you talking about, Father?"

"I mean this," he said with a sudden proud, almost haughty, air. "By Dharma, it is my duty to see that you marry properly. And what could be more proper than to marry a great Kuru lord? We are much honored by our lord's request. However, I must place a condition on this marriage, and when that condition is met, you both shall have all my blessings."

King Śan-tanu stared at the fisher king with surprise and suspicion. The Kuru lord's fiery eyes unnerved the fisher king, who struggled to regain his courage. He spoke quickly, before he again lost his nerve.

"O great Kuru king," he began, almost gasping, "like my daughter, you also speak truth, and never untruth. All the world honors you for that. So, I now ask that you promise me to accept my condition, and in return, my wife and I will give our blessings for this marriage."

Śan-tanu then said, "I shall hear your condition, fisher king, and then decide whether I shall comply. If you ask for that which may be given, I shall give it, otherwise not."

Śan-tanu glanced at Satya-vatī and she nodded her approval. Both knew the rules. They could only marry within the bounds of Dharma.

Satya-vatī had never seen Śan-tanu in this mood. He now spoke as a great king, not as a playful, fascinated suitor. But she dreaded her father's words, which were not long in coming.

He spoke to Śan-tanu in a voice that combined fulsome deference with coarse conceit. "O Kuru lord, Your Majesty, I am your humble servant."

Satya-vatī felt her stomach turning at this opening salvo, for she knew from Dāśa-rāja's tone and manner that bad things were coming. The proud fisherman continued, "I will joyfully and gratefully give my blessings to this most glorious union, if you will only deign to grant one simple request, which, as your most obedient servant, I place before you. I beg only that a son born to you and my precious daughter — my grandson — shall be your heir, the next Kuru king. My lord, that alone is my condition."

Satya's heart sank. She knew that even Śan-tanu himself could not rescind his son Deva-vrata's right to the throne, for Deva-vrata was already crown prince.

With a pained, apologetic look at Satya-vatī, Śan-tanu replied at once. "O fisher king, before I met your lovely daughter, I performed the ceremony of Yauva-rāja for my first son, Deva-vrata, born of the goddess Gaṅgā. By law, by Dharma, he is heir apparent and must inherit the Kuru throne. Even I cannot legally deny him, and even if I could, both honor and love forbid it, for I gave him my word."

When her so-called father dashed her hopes of happiness, and in so doing put the world at risk, Satya could not contain her anger. She trained her furious eyes on her foster father and said, "How can you do this to me? Why do you ruin my life? Withdraw your condition at once, if you love me."

Satya saw her foster father conceal the rage that rose within him when his so-called daughter thus addressed him, and in front of the Kuru king. But he could not hide it from Satya, who knew him too well. He bowed stiffly to Śan-tanu. "Forgive me, lord, but however my daughter may despise her own father, I act only with a father's love."

Satya saw Śan-tanu's anger. He was twice Dāśa-rāja's size and a legendary warrior. He could simply take her away at his will and the fisher king could do nothing. But she saw him calculating, even in his anger, and she knew that despite all his power, he would not take her under these circumstances.

He turned to Satya-vatī, and said, "Perhaps we can speak privately before I return to Hastinā-pura."

She agreed. He then faced the fisher king with cold civility and said, "I trust you will permit us to speak in private."

"Of course," came the prompt reply, accompanied by another bow.

Satya-vatī and Śan-tanu walked for the last time on the riverbank of sacred Yamunā. At first, they walked in silence. Satya begged the goddess to give her strength to endure this crushing disappointment.

Śan-tanu was first to speak. "Satya-vatī, I would take you away at once, regardless of what your father said, but as you know, that might ruin my reputation and yours. We are both servants of the people, and to protect them, we must have their trust. The world would accuse me of inducing you to break your vow to those people who raised you."

Heartbroken, Satya-vatī nodded in agreement as tears flowed down her cheeks. She said, "We live in dangerous times. If people lose faith in a Kuru king, they may be drawn away to Asuras, who will promise them anything. I understand that if we married and then revealed my royal parents, my foster parents would still create a public scandal, since they raised me. We already heard a sample of their attitude. They and their friends will shout to the world that they raised and loved me from birth, and that I swore a vow not to marry without their blessings. Looking back, I see that my foster father always resented my independent spirit. I spent over a year away with my real family. I now see how deeply the fisher king resented this. When I returned to the village a few months ago, he was especially bitter because I would not become a fisher like him, that instead of serving my foster parents, I faithfully served another couple in the Final Forest, even if they were the emperor and his wife. When I returned here after my parents departed, I could not bear this place, and my foster father certainly perceived that. All this time I was away, his resentment has been growing. I see that now. This explains his awful, stubborn interference in our marriage."

Crestfallen, Śan-tanu agreed. "Having met Dāśa-rāja, I see that you explained well his behavior. We know how the world would react to your breaking a vow to him, or to my inducing you to do so. People will censure our callous disregard for parents who sacrificed their lives for you, and so on. We both see the inevitable scandal."

"Yes, we do. My foster father would rouse the village, and thence it would spread far and wide, as scandal always does. The damage to your image, Śan-tanu, might be severe. It's not fair. It's not right. But it is real."

After many repetitions of their unbreakable love for each other, and as many reiterations of the insuperable obstacle to their union, Satya-vatī and Śan-tanu understood that the time had come to part.

He insisted that she keep the horse he secured for her. "I pray," he said, "it will always remind you of our happy times together."

She swore that it would. Through a veil of tears, Satya-vatī watched the man she loved ride away toward Hastina-pura. He turned several times to wave until the forest enveloped him, and she could see him no more. Too disturbed to speak with anyone, too depressed for any duty, she fled to her personal island and mourned the loss of Śan-tanu.

CHAPTER 25

She returned to the village in the dark of evening, desperate to avoid conversation with anyone. She heard a sound behind her and turned to see her foster parents approaching cautiously but steadily. She knew them well. They were determined to justify their actions before her.

Seeing them approach so confidently, Satya was disturbed beyond measure. Unable to control her anger, born of frustration, Satya-vatī shouted at the fisher king, "Why did you do this to me? Why did you ruin my life?"

"You don't know what is best for you. You've never known that. But I know."

"Absurd!" Satya shouted. "You don't know the harm you've caused to the world and to me!"

"What nonsense are you saying? What harm to the world?"

"You said strange animals have attacked sages. What if the animals are actually Asuras? Śan-tanu's son was born of a Devī. The Kurus and the world need him to rule. I am a human being. He is half Deva. His sons must be more powerful than mine."

These words startled the fisher king, but just for a moment. "That is all your imagination! Asura animals! No one has heard of such a thing. I acted for the best. You think I'm a nobody. But a very wise prince advised me. He came all the way here from a great kingdom to the east, one that is equal to the Kurus or anyone else. He came just to warn me. And he treated me like a king; he respected me! He revealed to me — most confidentially, of course, so don't tell anyone — that he has agents, spies everywhere, and that he knew a king would seek your hand in marriage. But this prince swore it was a trap, that the king who sought your hand, and his son, would mistreat and enslave you, and your future sons."

Satya's heart stopped with dread. "That is utter nonsense," she gasped. "Tell me, from what kingdom did that prince come?"

"Why do you care, Satya? Nothing I do matters to you."

"Father!" she cried, shocking Dāśa-rāja with her vehemence. "Tell me which prince came to you. Who was he? What did he tell you?"

Angry himself, the fisher king raised his voice. "He came from Magadha, and he said his name was Jarā-sandha."

"Oh my God!" Satya shouted. "Oh my God!"

"What is the matter with you?" Dāśa-rāja asked. "You should be proud that a great prince came all the way from Magadha to visit me. At least he respects me, even if my own daughter doesn't. He told me a mighty king would come here, seeking my daughter's hand, but that I should not consent unless the king swore that your son — *your* son, Satya-vatī — would be king. You saw that Śan-tanu couldn't promise that, even if he wanted to. His first son, Deva-vrata, will become king. Don't you see that? What will happen to you and my grandsons?"

"I'm sure Deva-vrata will be an excellent king," Satya shouted. "And he would have treated us very well."

"How can you be so naive?" Dāśa-rāja shouted. "Didn't you learn anything about politics when you spent all that time with the Cedi lords? Kings are jealous of their power. Since time began, a queen wants to see her son on the throne, not a stepson. Of course, your mother and I know that you would never plot against your own stepson. But your stepson will fear you. He must fear you, and his only safety will be to kill your son before he can grow up. Kill him, and seize his throne."

Satya flew into a rage. "What are you talking about? This is sheer madness! Did that demonic prince fill your mind with this poison?"

Dāśa-rāja had never seen such fury in his daughter. Unknown to him, she had strong warrior blood, toughened even further by the Devas for her special mission. He tried to calm her. But he was a very stubborn, unbending man. Seeing he could not console her, he grew impatient and insisted, "Say what you will. Śan-tanu's son will fear your sons and he will eliminate them. That's the danger of second marriages. I won't allow you to endanger my grandsons. If you are too good for us here, then marry a prince or king, but with no other heirs. That is my decision."

"So," she said angrily, "you must think there is a list of kings and princes seeking to marry me. That is nonsense! It was only Śan-tanu that wanted me, and you destroyed all my hopes."

Satya's heart beat rapidly. In anger she turned to Jarā-sandha, for whom she could not hide her contempt. "That prince, Jarā-sandha, is not a good man. He has no good intentions."

The fisher king made a puffing sound to show his disdain for her words. "You are wrong. He is a very nice prince. Why, his father is the great Bṛhad-ratha, son of Vasu, whom you so admired, indeed, whom you served so faithfully, when you should have served your own father. I thought you admired Bṛhad-ratha."

"I do, but the Magadha king does not hold his son Jarā-sandha in high esteem. I will appeal to Bṛhad-ratha, and he will tell you."

"Too late. I gave my word. You will not taint my honor again. You made us a laughingstock in our own village. Do you know that? You destroyed our hopes that you would stay with us."

His wife glanced plaintively at Satya. "Dāśa, don't be so hard on the girl. Satya, we love you, but you've humiliated your father long enough. He is only thinking of what's best for you. That Prince Jarā-sandha was kind enough to say that the world is a dangerous place. 'Your daughter will be safe only here, under your care.' He said those words himself."

Satya-vatī understood. Jarā-sandha had discovered her identity and conveyed a clear threat to her, one that her parents could never grasp or believe. If she left the region of this village, he might attack her. Jarā-sandha knew that Satya-vatī's marriage to Śan-tanu would forge a Kuru-Cedi alliance that would threaten the Asura mission. So, he took steps to block the marriage.

Desperate to be alone, to think, Satya excused herself as well as she could and flew to her boat. She raced to the island where her son was born, sat against an ancient tree, and brooded over her situation. She was not safe. She must find a way to send word to Matsya and her other brothers. But how could she reach them? The hot summer had begun and few travelers went down the river. Satya-vatī was trapped. She could flee to Śukti-matī, but she might only endanger her brothers and bring the Asura wrath upon them.

She thought of sending a message to Śan-tanu himself, but gave up the idea. He could not send Kuru troops to Cedi without provoking a dangerous international situation and possibly ruining any chance of a future Kuru-Cedi alliance. Satya had not given up all hope that her love would be fulfilled, along with the alliance.

She had her horse, whom she named Vāyu-ja, Born of the Wind, and a little boat. Perhaps she could find shelter in Hastinā-pura. No, the humiliation of going there and being rejected (a real possibility) would be far worse than death.

Under a bright full moon, she stayed for an hour on her secluded isle, and the next day rode Vāyu-ja deep into the woods. She avoided the brāhmaṇa village, fearing that she might bring the Asuras there.

She thought of calling her son, Dvaipāyana, but this might place him in danger. If Jarā-sandha knew her identity, he probably also knew of the young Avatāra. Indeed, the Asura's plan might be to induce or pressure her to summon the Avatāra, to thus draw him into a trap and attack him. She could not risk that now.

She thought of praying for Parā-śara to return. His image in her mind reassured her. He foretold her marriage to a great king. But he had not given her a means to call him. He might not even be in this universe. She knew that his promise would come true only if she did not die now at the hands of her nephew Jarā-sandha, or his agents.

The mighty Asura himself came all the way to her village to sabotage her marriage to Śan-tanu. He and his Asura agents might appear anywhere. She must ever be on guard. But how could she defend herself? If only her foster father could grasp the danger he put her in. In his misguided attempt to promote what he perceived to be the family interest, he had deprived her of her true protector, Śan-tanu, and placed her in great danger.

Another danger presented itself. Several minutes after the mighty Kuru king departed, Dāśa-rāja suddenly realized what he had done. He had refused his daughter's hand to the most powerful man in the world, and in doing so, had clearly implied that Śan-tanu's first son, Deva-vrata, was not to be trusted, or worse, was potentially evil. The fisher king now realized to his horror that he had deeply insulted the most powerful man on Earth, a man who could quite easily arrange the fisherman's death.

Dāśa-rāja revealed his fears to his foster daughter, who at first took pains to assure him that Śan-tanu was a virtuous king who would not do such a thing. But then her confidence failed her. She had seen Śan-tanu almost exclusively in relaxed, informal situations, latterly when he was courting her favor. And she now recalled that when her foster father denied him her hand, the Kuru monarch had shown, even if subtly, a proud, angry air that she had never seen in him before.

Of his son, Deva-vrata, she knew almost nothing. Naturally, a loving father would attribute many virtues to a faithful son. But in his anger and frustration,

Śan-tanu might reveal to his son the extremely disparaging insinuations that the fisher king made about Deva-vrata, the heir apparent to the Kuru throne. Deva-vrata was still a young adolescent, but all reports indicated that the prince, born of a goddess and a Kuru lord, wielded terrible power.

Brooding over the situation, Satya considered it possible that the Kuru prince would take the fisher king's words as a personal offense, an offense greatly magnified by the pain and humiliation caused to a beloved father. The prince might then impulsively ride straight to the fishing village to avenge the offense to his father, to himself, and indeed to his proud Kuru dynasty.

When both had calmed their tempers enough to actually speak to each other, her foster father revealed to Satya-vatī that he shared her fears. Satya longed to trust Śan-tanu's virtuous nature, but after repeatedly analyzing possibilities and probabilities, she found herself dreading that her brief association with the Kuru king would cause the death of her foster father.

CHAPTER 26

Weeks passed, and neither Śan-tanu personally, nor his son or agents, came to wreak revenge on the fisher king. Satya understood. Śan-tanu was honorable, as she believed. But he sent no message to her. Their relationship was over. Their mutual love would gradually lapse into a memory, soon to be erased when Śan-tanu found an equal, but less complicated, match.

Having returned to glorious Hastinā-pura, he was again surrounded by imperial splendor. News came from all sides that the Kuru king was increasingly hailed as Earth's leading monarch. The loveliest princesses must be vying for his hand. It could not be otherwise.

How ironic that Satya's brief, romantic encounter with Śan-tanu did not lead to their marriage, but did free him from his grief over Gaṅgā, thus enabling him to marry another princess.

Satya-vatī could not shake off her depression. For a few precious moments, she had dared to hope she had found the love of her life, only to watch helplessly as her own so-called father ruined those hopes forever.

Much as she feared for her foster father's life, she could not give up her bitter anger toward him, for even now he insisted he had done the right thing. Now, even more than when she first returned from her joyful reunion with her real family, she found it impossible to stay in the fishing village. Everything here reminded her of what she had lost — a divine son, and an ideal husband. Indeed, her conviction that she and Śan-tanu were perfectly matched only increased when all hope of their union was gone.

She must leave this village, and she hardly cared anymore if Jarā-sandha killed her. A new life in a new body might be best. She would not reveal to her foster parents that her departure was permanent, for she feared what they would say, and even more, what she would say in reply. So, she told them that she was going for some time. She did not lie. In this mortal world, any amount of time was but some time. They did not protest or argue, having given up any hope that she would be like she was before.

Thus, one day, at the first reddish streaks of dawn, Satya-vatī made her way downstream in her little boat (she had no strength to row upstream). Her devoted horse, Vāyu-ja, happily followed her along the riverbank. As she floated down dear Yamunā, she rebuked herself for heading straight to the last place where she and Śan-tanu had been carefree and happy together, laughing together as she bested him in a race across the river. Her own mind called her a fool for helplessly steering her boat straight to that last happy place.

She arrived and sat on the riverbank as Vāyu-ja grazed. Cool breezes skimmed her skin and ruffled her hair. Spirits downcast, she stared into Yamunā's unending waters. The sun briefly emerged from behind dark clouds and made the water glitter, only to vanish again.

Satya-vatī knew not how long she sat there without aim or energy, brooding over past events and crushed hopes. As night swallowed the light, she lay down on the grassy bank, without will or reason to seek greater comfort or shelter.

Dawn opened her eyes, but could not rouse her heart. She found no reason to stay or go, to sit or stand, to eat or fast. Tired of life itself, she lay back down on the riverbank. But her son, Dvaipāyana, entered her mind. She realized she could not abandon life. Parā-śara entered her mind, as real as when they sat together in the brāhmaṇa village. He repeated his promise, urged her to believe him, and then vanished from her mind.

Satya-vatī sat up straight, crossed her legs in a yoga āsana, greeted the river goddess, and chose hope and life. Suddenly, she heard the two-beat trot of approaching horses, their hooves clapping the Earth in military synchrony. The sound grew louder. It came from the north, raising dust clouds that drifted above the trees.

A contingent of cavalry burst into view, flying on high-stepping steeds, and heading straight toward her. Satya-vatī folded her arms across her chest defiantly. If they were her nephew Jarā-sandha's assassins, or if that young Asura himself had come, she would die proudly, fearlessly, cursing them with her last breath. She would die like the worthy daughter of an emperor.

As they came near, she was astonished to see that these men bore the proud colors and emblems of the mighty Kurus. Had they come to take her away to Śan-tanu? Or to take vengeance on her foster father?

Trembling in anticipation, she relaxed her arms and waited. They reached her in moments and dismounted. A middle-aged man dressed in the smart uniform of a royal minister approached her, followed by a large youth, whose dress, ensign, and symbols marked him beyond doubt as a Kuru prince. He could not be more than fifteen or sixteen years old, yet his body was tall, and exuded power.

Both men greeted her respectfully. Satya-vatī honored them in turn with a curt bow. The prince then said in a clear, confident, respectful tone, "Greetings, good lady. I am Deva-vrata, son of Śan-tanu, our Kuru lord. We come from Hastinā-pura, seeking an audience with the honorable Satya-vatī. Kindly tell me if you are that good lady, or if not, where we can find her."

Trying to appear calm, she said, "I am Satya-vatī. I hope that you, prince, and your companions, traveled well from your great capital."

Deva-vrata smiled and bowed his head. "Thank you for your kind concern. We traveled well. Let me introduce Śarma, a trusted advisor to my father, the king."

The older man stepped forward, bowed to Satya-vatī, and stood at relaxed attention, discreetly studying her. Satya politely returned his bow. "I am honored by your visit, sirs. I can offer little in the way of hospitality, but I will gladly bring pure river water, or provide you with fruits and nuts. Simple forest fare is all I can offer you."

Graciously declining this offer, Deva-vrata and Śarma requested Satya-vatī grant them a private meeting, to discuss relevant topics. She promptly agreed.

Śarma asked the soldiers to find a secluded place to bathe and eat their rations. Satya sat with the two men by the river. After a brief silence, Śarma gave the prince a look, indicating that he must speak. The prince nodded and said, "Satya-vatī, with your permission, I will briefly explain certain events in my life that have ultimately brought me here today."

Satya assured Deva-vrata that she was most eager to hear anything that the prince wished to tell her. His earnest smile showed how much her words encouraged him.

He began. "My father must have told you that my mother, Gaṅgā Devī, took me to the Deva world soon after my birth. She raised me there."

"Yes, he did tell me. Indeed, all the world knows that."

"Indeed. Well, four years ago, when I was twelve years old, my mother brought me to my father. I was destined to spend this life in the human world."

Satya nodded with compassion. "So, that means you are now only sixteen years old."

"Yes, sixteen."

Satya sighed. "So, for the first twelve years of your life, you didn't know your father."

"Correct. But my mother did tell me about him, and I wanted more than anything to meet him. I thought of him constantly. I dreamed of meeting him. I wondered, what would he think of me? Would he be proud of me? When I finally returned, my father welcomed me with so much love and joy. He has been a perfect father to me."

"You are most fortunate to have such a father," Satya said, feeling more than ever what she had lost in Śan-tanu, and comparing him with her foster father.

"Yes, I am most fortunate. But I also suffered, because I saw that in all those years, my father had never gotten over losing my mother. He could not forget that Gaṅgā had been his wife, and was the mother of his only son. For my sake, he struggled to conceal his pain. But I saw that his broken heart did not heal. For four years, I've watched a most beloved father's suffering."

Deva-vrata looked down sadly. Feeling his pain, Satya-vatī said quietly, "I can easily imagine how difficult that must be." Śarma's stoic expression could not conceal his own pain at the king's misery. Satya began to doubt that Śan-tanu could ever love again, after losing such a goddess.

But how could his sad narration lead to Satya's union with Śan-tanu? Why had the prince come at all? Deva-vrata looked up and answered her question.

"Noble lady," he said, "I explained all this to you, because when my father returned recently, we found his mood to be quite changed. He no longer lamented for Gaṅgā. He had fallen deeply in love with you. He personally told me that only you had the power to heal his broken heart. Then he lost you, because your foster father would only give his consent if your future son became the Kuru king."

Deva-vrata's confirmation of Śan-tanu's continuing deep love for her, beyond what she had dared imagine possible, deeply affected her. Her anger returned, though she hid it, over the ignorant, cruel condition her foster father had placed on the union. She saw that Deva-vrata seemed to be waiting for her response, which she now gave. "All that you said about my foster father's interference is true. I am ashamed of what he did. And I grieve for noble Śan-tanu." And for myself, she thought.

Hearing this, Deva-vrata glanced at Śarma, who nodded to the prince, as if resigned to a previously agreed-upon plan. The prince then said, "Forgive me, but when I discovered what your foster father had done, I was furious. I shouted to the ministers that great Śan-tanu is the most powerful man in the world. Why should he care what a fisherman says? Śarma, please tell Satya-vatī what you said to me in reply."

The royal advisor nodded. "I and the other counselors simply explained that we are Kurus, not Asuras. We serve the sacred Law, and thereby serve all the citizens. Justice is our power. In order to protect and serve the innocent, your noble father, Śan-tanu, acts with unrivaled courage and power. But he will never impose his will for personal pleasure, or happiness."

This account fully confirmed Satya's own conviction of Śan-tanu's excellent character. She was proud of him. Never had she felt so strongly as now that Śan-tanu was the ideal man for her. She grieved for having ever suggested that she and Śan-tanu stop by the fishing village, and for having agreed not to marry without her foster father's blessings. She had made a terrible blunder. But she had given her word and could not retract it. Neither her sense of honor nor Śan-tanu's would allow them to marry. So, why had Deva-vrata come?

Sunk in these thoughts, she took a moment to realize that Deva-vrata was addressing her. He said, "Noble lady, I have one last question, which I shall ask with your permission."

"Of course," she replied. "You may ask anything."

"Thank you. Forgive my candor, but I must know. Do you love my father as truly as he loves you?"

Satya colored at this blunt question. Yet, no graceful, oblique reply came to her mind. The prince's simple, sincere query demanded a simple, sincere reply. She gave one. "Yes, I do love him, just as he loves me."

Deva-vrata smiled and glanced at Śarma. The counselor nodded stoically. The prince then said to Satya-vatī, "Noble lady, clearly, I am the only person on Earth that can end my father's misery. By Dharma, I was anointed into yauva-rājya, the status of heir apparent. Therefore, by Law, by Dharma, no one else can deny me, or claim for another, the Kuru throne, when my father ends his tenure."

"Yes, everyone knows of your good fortune," Satya said, fearing what he would say next.

"But I have the right to renounce my claim, in favor of your future son, and that is precisely what I came to do."

"You cannot do that!" Satya-vatī cried, startling Deva-vrata and Śarma with her vehemence. Silence ensued, since clearly, Satya's reaction had not entered into the men's calculations, and they were not sure what to say. Satya's heart was breaking, for though she wanted more than anything to marry Śan-tanu, she could not betray her honor and duty by trading the happiness of an innocent prince for her own.

Torn by strong emotions, Satya-vatī insisted, "O prince, I honor you more than I can express for your selfless wish to give up so much for a beloved father. But I cannot, I will not, let you do so. You would suffer future misery that, as a youth, you cannot now imagine. You have no idea of the needs and feelings of a mature man, nor how you will suffer if I allow you to carry out this plan. Your wise counselor Śarma must know exactly what I mean."

She glanced at Śarma, and he nodded his agreement. But clearly, he had no power to convince the prince.

Deva-vrata insisted that he grew up on Deva-loka, a higher world than Earth, and this planet did not tempt or gratify him. "So you see," he said, "my sacrifice is not so great. Having experienced both worlds, I seek, ultimately, the World Beyond. My vow will be a type of yoga practice."

Satya-vatī protested, "I respect your ideals and your character, but do you really claim to be free of all attachment?"

"Maybe not," he said. "Perhaps I am still attached to the glory of keeping my vows. That, in my view, is an even higher personal power than that of the warrior."

"True, but attachment to personal power, high or low, can still bind one to this mortal world."

A doubt seemed to flicker in Deva-vrata's eyes, but he rejected it and said, "Forgive me, but I must do this for my father."

A terrible thought crossed Satya-vatī's mind. What if Śan-tanu had ordered his son to renounce the throne? That would be disgraceful. She was sure Śan-tanu would never do that, but she must confirm it. She turned to Deva-vrata. "O Prince, tell me, please, does your father know of your plan? Does he even know that you came here?"

Deva-vrata looked down. "No, he does not know." Śarma nodded in confirmation. Satya saw that he was a serious brāhmaṇa who could not lie. Śan-tanu was innocent. Satya-vatī was now determined that Deva-vrata not sacrifice his future for hers. He was noble, sincere, but too young to grasp what he was doing.

But what of the desperately needed Kuru-Cedi alliance? She told herself that even if she did not marry Śan-tanu, she would go to him in Hastinā-pura, put aside her pride and dignity, and beg him to form an alliance with her brothers. He was a good and just king and would respond to objective moral authority. He still loved her, and for her sake and the good of the world, he would do the right thing.

With an aching heart, Satya-vatī was about to declare her final decision not to marry the Kuru king under these circumstances. But before she could speak, Deva-vrata cried out, "Dear lady, I shall not condemn my father to a lifetime of grief. He loves you with all his heart. I must do this."

Alarmed, Satya-vatī shouted, "Deva-vrata, you took birth in this world to protect it from Asuras. Do not give up your power to do so!" But even as she spoke these words, she thought, Is Deva-vrata truly on our side? Would he fight the Asuras? Desperate to find out, she said, "Your father is devoted to Viṣṇu. Do you share that devotion? I ask because, if you do, I'm sure that you would only renounce your throne if you were *fully* convinced that by doing so, you would please Viṣṇu."

Her words startled him. She anxiously awaited his answer.

He replied, "I do share my father's devotion to Viṣṇu. I had not thought about this particular case, but I believe Viṣṇu will accept my decision and my service."

She appreciated, but could not support, his immature reasoning. His was a youthful devotion, lacking the mature consideration of his father. Before she could speak again, he declared, "Kind lady, I will not turn back from my decision. I shall bring happiness to my father and king! Please tell me that you will not reject my father and thus render my sacrifice useless."

"Of course I would not do that. I love your father, but—"

Before she could finish, Deva-vrata jumped to his feet, bowed to her, and gave a powerful blast on his conch. The Kuru soldiers came running, bringing the horses. Satya jumped to her feet. But the two men were already hurrying to their mounts. The soldiers had already mounted.

Satya ran after them, pleading with them to wait. They profusely apologized, the prince signaled his royal guards, and the entire Kuru contingent rode swiftly away, Deva-vrata outpacing the others.

Satya-vatī cried out in exasperation, and threw her hands in the air. She sat by the river, torn by conflicting emotions. She had tried with all her heart to stop Deva-vrata from renouncing his throne. If, despite her efforts, he did renounce, she would blamelessly marry Śan-tanu. This prospect moved her, despite her best efforts at self-abnegation.

A moment later another thought entered her mind and sent a chill up her spine. She had tested Deva-vrata and found him to possess, in regard to Viṣṇu, at least the unschooled devotion of an adolescent. But what of Satya's own eldest son, yet to be born? What if he, like her brother Bṛhad-ratha's eldest son, turned out to be an Asura? Even Indra himself could not stop Jarā-sandha from entering the womb of her brother's wife. If Deva-vrata renounced, and her own son was an Asura, her son would take control of the Kuru dynasty. If Deva-vrata remained loyal to his Kuru dynasty, he would be forced to serve that Asura. Jarā-sandha would then rule the Cedis, and an Asura ally would rule the mighty Kurus. The world would be lost. She trembled at this thought. She must stop Deva-vrata.

Satya jumped to her feet, threw her few possessions into a bag, and frantically ran about, searching for Vāyu-ja, whom she found grazing in the woods. She cried out, and he trotted to her.

Breathless, she threw herself on his back, and sent him galloping after the Kuru prince. She must reach her father before Deva-vrata resigned his throne and ruined his life!

CHAPTER 27

Desperate to catch up with Deva-vrata, Satya entreated Vāyu-ja to go faster. But the Kuru prince had the power of a Deva, and his horse flew like the wind.

Satya raced through meadows, bounded over fallen trees, and splashed through streams, fearing she was falling ever farther behind that son of a goddess. Panting and breathless, horse and rider arrived at her eerily quiet village. Tension hung thick in the air. Deva-vrata sat huddled with Counselor Śarma near the river. Dāśa-rāja moved about confidently, speaking softly to the village elders. His wife stood in the middle of a group of ladies, gesturing with both hands.

Satya left Vāyu-ja to drink and bathe in the river. For a moment, she stood, hands on hips, surveying the scene. No one but Dāśa-rāja looked happy. Only he smiled.

Śarma turned his head and saw her. His downcast face alarmed her. He stood and came to her, asking if they could speak privately. She led him to a private area by the river and they sat on a wooden bench.

The counselor was sad. "It is all settled. Deva-vrata has renounced the Kuru throne. I am happy for you and the king. Truly, I am. But..."

Śarma's voice choked, and tears welled in his eyes. He composed himself and said, "But the prince...he does not understand what he is doing. Later, he will suffer. And, with all respect to your future sons, the kingdom will suffer, more than anyone can imagine."

Satya-vatī could think of nothing to say. A full minute passed. The counselor turned to her with an anguished expression. "Our meeting with Dāśa-rāja was terrible. Far worse than I imagined possible."

"What do you mean?" cried Satya-vatī. "How could it be worse? I beg you, tell me at once."

"Our encounter began as I expected. The fisher king received us well, externally. He observed the rules of hospitality, and honored the prince with words and gifts, humble as they were. Deva-vrata and I then sat with him and the village elders sat around us."

Satya-vatī said, "I can just imagine. Then what?"

Counselor Śarma explained that Dāśa-rāja continued to praise the prince, slyly adding that the prince was so powerful, that anyone who ran afoul of him would be in grave danger. Thus, Dāśa-rāja claimed to fear for the lives of his royal grandsons, if Satya-vatī married the Kuru king.

Deva-vrata took this as an attack on his character. He angrily said, "Sir, do you attack my honor? Do you think me so devoid of decency that, having renounced the throne, I would harm a younger brother who rightfully claimed it? If you, sir, now declare me capable of such evil, you will pay for your offense."

At this, all the fisher elders cried out to the prince to spare Dāśa-rāja's life. They knew the prince's power, and urged their king not to offend him.

The fisher king then begged the prince not to misunderstand him. "I am but a loving father, anxious, like all fathers, to do all he can to protect his daughter. I am a humble man. How could I know the exact character of an exalted Kuru prince? Believe me, I do not accuse you, but I do not know you. I beg you, allow me to act as a loving father who means no offense to you. My only concern was my grandson's safety. I have no other concern. Your father is the best husband for my daughter. Forgive me!"

Though distrusting Dāśa-rāja's motives, Deva-vrata controlled his anger, for his father's sake. "I vowed," Deva-vrata said angrily, "that I would bring the honorable maiden Satya-vatī to my father. I shall keep my vow."

The counselor groaned. "The condition demanded of Śan-tanu was repeated to Deva-vrata, who then formally renounced the Kuru throne in favor of your son. I was devastated. The prince was glad for his father. Deva-vrata and I believed the matter settled. We felt most uncomfortable in this village, as you can imagine, and we were anxious to find you and depart for Hastinā-pura. But then, the fisher king, without warning, insisted on two additional vows."

Satya's heart sank. "Two more vows! What could they be?"

Śarma leaned back and sighed. He put his fingers on his forehead, and ran them through his hair. Eyes closed, he shook his head slowly and explained what took place.

The fisher king said, "Dear prince, you acted with true love for your father, and I honor your vow. I would never doubt your excellent character. But, Your Highness, there is but one more issue..." His voice trailed off, as if fearing the prince's anger.

"What are you getting at?" Śarma demanded. "Speak plainly."

"Of course," the fisher king said with a bow. "As I said, I do not doubt the noble prince. But...the prince might have a son. And there lies a great doubt."

"Do not try my patience," the prince warned angrily. "You heard the counselor. Speak plainly!"

Dāśa-rāja bowed low and said, "My lords, no father can assume that his son will inherit all the father's excellent qualities. Indeed, in cases like these, my prince, your son may well resent that you gave up your throne to a younger stepbrother, thus depriving your son of that throne. It would be only too human for your son, Your Majesty, to deeply resent his fate, and to see his cousin — my grandson — as a villain. Your son might be sorely tempted to right what he sees as a terrible wrong, and this would put my poor grandson in grave danger. Surely, history shows that such things happen."

Counselor Śarma, who had been narrating these events to Satya-vatī, now paused, looked at her, and said, "I'm sure you can see the terrible trap that your foster father had laid for my prince."

Satya's eyes opened wide in alarm. She saw the trap. And it was grotesque and cruel. Dāśa-rāja first coerced the prince to renounce his lawful throne, clearly implying, though never explicitly stating, that he would then give his daughter to Śan-tanu. Once Deva-vrata gave up his throne, and could not take it back, the scheming fisher king then demanded a second condition — that Deva-vrata agree to never marry and have children, to spend the rest of his life alone.

When Śarma confirmed Satya-vatī's surmise, she gasped, and tears filled her eyes. She knew from Śarma that Deva-vrata never broke his vows, no matter the consequences. He was quite headstrong in such matters.

Satya-vatī cried out, "How awful! The prince had already given up his throne, yet my father would not bestow me on Śan-tanu until the prince granted another outrageous request. So unless Deva-vrata complied, he would still lose the throne, and not win my hand for his father. The ancient Kuru lineage would be thrown into chaos." Satya trembled in rage at this unholy machination.

With his head in his hands, Śarma said, "And there was yet a third condition."

Furious at her foster father, Satya-vatī insisted that Śarma explain at once this third condition. It was this: for the rest of his life, Deva-vrata would only take up weapons at the explicit behest of a reigning Kuru monarch. And he could not refuse such a request. The fisher king had cited the case of his own late and lamented King Vasu, to use his words. As we all know, though born a Kuru, Vasu gained control of the Cedi kingdom, and expanded it into an empire. Deva-vrata could just as easily leave the Kurus, and conquer any kingdom he liked. He could then march upon Hastinā-pura. Who could oppose him? At his whim, Deva-vrata could subjugate the Kurus, and bring them under his power, though technically acting as the king of a foreign state."

"Surely your prince would never contemplate such evil!" Satya-vatī cried.

"Certainly not! But this dark, insolent demand seemed rational to its author, Dāśa-rāja."

Thus Deva-vrata vowed to take up arms only and always at the order, and under the command, of a lawful Kuru monarch. So, Deva-vrata could never fight against the Kurus of Hastinā-pura, or rule and defend another realm. And he *must* fight at the command of a Kuru monarch. Though this third demand further offended his character, the prince had no choice but to comply. Satya-vatī could not imagine how the mighty prince, son of a Kuru king and a goddess, could bear such blasphemous insinuations.

As if grasping and sharing her thoughts, the minister lamented, "God knows I tried to dissuade the prince. But of course, I could not. I have always yearned and prayed for my lord, Śan-tanu, to be happy. But this comes at too great a cost. And how will the king be happy knowing what his son has lost? The prince is too young to consider these things. On hearing these terrible vows, the Devas, who closely monitored these events, and who knew Deva-vrata from his infancy, cried out, 'Bhīṣma! Frightful!' And now the villagers, taking the Deva utterance as high praise, call him Bhīṣma!"

Satya-vatī realized with a shudder that the Devas had cried out bhīṣma with good reason. Deva-vrata's vow was not only frightful in its self-inflicted severity; the mighty prince had also renounced his authority to initiate resistance against the Asuras. For the rest of his life, the new Bhīṣma could only defend Earth from Asuras if the Kuru king, whoever that might be in the future, chose to engage him thus. A mighty Asura had already taken birth in the august Cedi line, and even Indra could not stop him. Were an Asura to someday inherit the Kuru throne, Bhīṣma's vow would force him to fight on the Asura side, to fight for evil.

"Oh God help us!" Satya cried out. "The prince does not know what he has done."

"No, he does not," Śarma said. "And now, even his own soldiers call him Bhīṣma, taking it as a high compliment to their prince, since the Devas first uttered the name. The world has gone mad."

Counselor Śarma finished his narration. Grasping the full barbarity of Dāśa-rāja's intrigue, Satya-vatī went looking for Deva-vrata. She found the prince walking and brooding in the surrounding woods, his hands clasped behind his back, eyes fixed on the ground.

Satya-vatī rustled the grass as she walked to avoid startling him. He saw her coming and folded his hands in respectful salute. She quickly returned the courtesy and asked if they could talk. He was happy to speak to her on any topic she chose. They sat together on soft grass under an ancient tree. She told him at once how ashamed she was of her foster father's actions, and how deeply she regretted the demands imposed upon the prince.

Her words brought a grateful smile to his lips, but he assured her that he was sincerely happy to make any sacrifice for the father he adored. She praised him for his devotion, but her expression clearly showed that she continued to lament his fate.

He again insisted that, having grown up on Deva-loka, he felt little attachment to the powers and riches of Earth. Indeed, having lived in both worlds, he now aspired to the World Beyond as the only place of true and lasting happiness. This reminded her of what her parents had taught her in the Final Forest. But Vasu and Girikā were ending their life. Bhīṣma, as everyone now called Deva-vrata, was just beginning his.

Seeing her incredulity, Bhīṣma again tried to persuade her not to lament his fate. He insisted he was content with his fate. He now saw his life as yoga, a spiritual practice of detachment and equanimity in all circumstances.

Satya-vatī exclaimed, "O brave prince, when you are older, you will see what you have done, and what you have lost. Forgive my bold words, but I feel for you. You have stated that you may be attached to the power of keeping your vows. But attachment to Viṣṇu is even higher. That attachment alone can safely lead us to the World Beyond."

Her words struck him. After deep thought, he nodded, evidently pleased with her devotion to Viṣṇu. Satya did not belabor her point. Few human beings could focus exclusively on the highest spiritual attainments. The glory of serving his father, and keeping his vows, was all the worldly dignity left to the young prince. She would not cruelly deprive him of it. Instead, she assured him of her genuine admiration and support, and urged him to take her at once to Hastinā-pura. It would be his pleasure.

She could not bear to remain in the fishing village with a parent who had fallen so low in her eyes, but she must take her leave in a proper way. She would always be grateful to her foster parents for raising her. She would always love them for having loved her. Yet, to preserve that gratitude and love, she must leave at once. She found her parents in their cottage, looking as if they expected her.

CHAPTER 28

Satya-vatī entered the modest thatched cottage that had been her home for so long. In this dwelling, her mother had fed and nurtured her, her father had protected her.

This lifelong home now oppressed and angered her. A complete picture assembled itself in her mind. Her real parents, as she now realized, had regularly sent funds to Dāśa-rāja, but he hoarded it, and always claimed to be in need. With this money, he had begun to think highly of himself, and dreamed of a more respectable life. It pained her to see clearly her foster father's weaknesses. And she could not overcome her anger for what he had done to Deva-vrata. That anger pressed her to say heavy things to the fisher king.

But she would only make things worse by offending or wounding those who raised her, those who believed she was theirs to bestow in marriage. She entered the cottage but remained standing. Her father quickly provoked her. "So, girl, I have done all this for our family. You will be a great queen. It is all for the best. I am proud of you, and of myself."

Satya-vatī struggled to conceal her rage and frustration. She had been willing to suffer the heartbreak of losing Śan-tanu. She would then have gone to Hastinā-pura and begged him to form an alliance with her brothers. She believed that his love for her, and his honor and intelligence, would have induced him to grant her appeal.

But now! She could not bear to see her foster father rob a noble young prince of his life, and then brag about it. Never had she been so disgusted. Desperate to leave, to escape, she restrained her rage and spoke the few proper, polite words they expected from her.

But as she turned to leave, something in her heart rebelled, and forced these words from her lips: "You must see that, whatever your motives, you have destroyed the life of a kind and innocent prince!" She knew her foster parents would react, and they did.

"Do not attack us!" her mother cried. "We love you. We raised you. We are simple, ignorant people who did their best for you. I beg you, do not hate us! I could not bear that. I pray the Devas bless you to be happy. Can't you pray for our happiness? Leave us in love, not in hatred."

These words affected Satya deeply. She stood motionless, unable to stop the tears that ran down her cheeks. "I can never hate you," she said softly. "I love you for all you have done for me, and I will never forget."

At these words, her foster mother burst into tears. When her loud sobs quieted, Satya said, "Please do not think me an evil child. I am not. But there are forces that threaten our world. You need not worry about that. But as a queen, I will have important new duties. Just as you did your duty as best you could, so must I. And to do my duty, I must ask Father a question that he may not like. But I beg you both, do not blame me for asking it. We are all trying our best to follow our Dharma."

"You may ask me anything," Dāśa-rāja said, moved by her words.

"Thank you. Father, before you agreed to my marriage with Śan-tanu, you made his son vow to accept three conditions."

"Yes, I did."

"Did the Magadha prince, Jarā-sandha, play any role in this? Did he advise you or influence you to make your three demands? I must know."

"Young lady," he said with some agitation, "you told me that Jarā-sandha is not a good man. I believed you. I did not speak with him again. In this case, I myself decided on those three demands. And I'm proud of them. The Devas know I don't want to hurt anyone, but my family comes first. Not some prince, whoever he may be."

Satya knew that Dāśa-rāja had always coveted a high connection for his family, especially his future grandson. He claimed it was all for his daughter, but Satya-vatī knew that his ambition, his lust for prestige, drove him to ruin Deva-vrata's life.

Satya wanted to shout at him, *You had no need to exact these crazy vows! Why didn't you just trust the prince? His father is noble Śan-tanu! For God's sake, his mother is a goddess, but you couldn't trust him! What is wrong with you?*

But this fiery rebuke from a young daughter would bring nothing but an irreparable rupture. Even now, Dāśa-rāja fell silent, his guilty face revealing that he knew all that Satya wanted to say. He said nothing, for his daughter's demeanor wakened him to the reality that he had indeed offended a most powerful prince. Hearing what the fisher had done to his son, Śan-tanu himself might seek revenge. And the fisher's own daughter, Satya, would be a powerful queen, capable of persuading her husband to do her will. Thus, Dāśa-rāja prudently sought to leave his daughter — for she would depart soon — on good terms. Satya-vatī read his thoughts. Thus, with very different motives, father and daughter played their parts well, each determined to part in apparent mutual good will.

Satya-vatī invited her foster parents to the wedding, and as she fully expected, and wanted, they declined. "It would be such a great honor," her mother said, "but forgive us, we are too old to travel so far. And our crude manners would only embarrass you."

Satya-vatī protested against this, but her father insisted that people would laugh at them in that sophisticated city. "Hastinā-pura is even grander than our Cedi capital. This village is our home. Forgive us."

Having no wish to dissuade them, Satya quietly acquiesced. She had one last request. She begged her foster parents not to speak to anyone outside the village about her marriage, and to order the other village residents to follow the same rule. It was extremely important to Satya-vatī that her dear brothers hear about this first from her, and not from public rumor and gossip. Satya-vatī had no way, at present, to communicate with them. The Kurus would find it suspicious if she requested that Kuru envoys communicate to the Cedi rulers before the official Kuru announcements of the event. Generally, the Kurus would take offense at a fisherman and his cohort usurping the right of the Kurus to make the marriage public. Even more troubling, Śan-tanu had not yet agreed to his son's arrangement on his behalf. Śan-tanu had made it clear that Deva-vrata's ascension to the throne was a condition of their marriage. Now that condition had been irrevocably violated. This filled Satya-vatī with dread.

Further, possible Kuru displeasure with the prince's arrangement would be seriously exacerbated if the Kurus discovered that news of a wedding, not yet agreed to by their king, was being spread around the world from a fishing village.

Thus, it was imperative that news not yet spread around the world of her upcoming marriage. Her foster parents saw no harm in letting the fishers talk about the wedding, and thus letting the news spread. Dāśa-rāja was anxious to bask in the prestige of a royal connection.

But Satya-vatī insisted so vehemently that he must wait until the Kurus announced the event, and that this was the necessary etiquette, that he finally agreed to this rule. Satya had no idea how strenuously he would enforce it.

It was time to leave. Her foster parents blessed her, and prayed to the Devas to bless her. Dāśa-rāja said, "Remember us now and then, and kindly forgive our mistakes."

In reply, Satya-vatī said all the right things, and bowed to them. Within minutes, she was amazed to find herself sitting in a royal Kuru carriage, resplendent with the colors and crest of the mighty dynasty. She was headed to the grandest of earthly cities, though not without considerable anxiety.

Counselor Śarma sat facing her. Bhīṣma, heavily armed, rode by their side. Satya's horse, Vāyu-ja, trotted behind them. With a shout from a cavalry commander, a Kuru platoon, with perfect precision, surrounded the carriage. As its wheels began to turn, all the fishing community cheered, and begged the Devas to bless the trip. The journey to Hastinā-pura had begun.

When they were well beyond the Kalpi area, Counselor Śarma said, "We are sending royal messengers to inform kingdoms along the way of our coming, and to carry the prince's personal message to his father. Is there anyone to whom we can send a message from you?"

This question reminded her that she must communicate all the recent events to her brothers. But how? Messages were only sent by spoken word, through messengers with prodigious memories. She believed that royal Kuru messengers were most discreet, yet she could not bring herself to reveal to a herald, or even to her brothers, the mortifying situation in which she found herself. She was traveling to Hastinā-pura, perhaps to be humiliated on an unprecedented global scale, if Śan-tanu rejected her. How could he form an alliance with a family whose elders had ruined his son's life?

Only if and when accepted by, and properly betrothed to, Śan-tanu, who had not yet accepted her under these new circumstances, could she reveal everything to her brothers. Even if a rumor about this affair reached them, by that time, she would have arrived in the Kuru land, and she would know Śan-tanu's decision. She would then have ample time to explain everything to her brothers.

"Thank you for your kind offer," she replied to Śarma, "but at this time I have no message to send."

Śarma then asked sincerely if the Kurus could do anything to make her travel more pleasant, less wearisome or anxious. Satya-vatī thanked him, praising the kindness of her hosts. She had all she could possibly need or desire.

Śarma then explained that their initial route would take them northwest along the Yamunā River. They would stop that night precisely at the point where their path turned to the north, away from the river. Both Śarma and Deva-vrata were anxious to afford Satya a last evening on the bank of the river, since they had heard from the king that she was devoted to Yamunā. This genuine concern for her feelings moved her.

Śarma added that when they stopped, he and the prince wanted to explain to her some important details of their trip. Satya-vatī nodded, wondering anxiously what the important details could be.

As the party moved northwest along the silvery banks of Yamunā, the rhythmic clack of steady-stepping horses gave a sweet cadence to their journey. Delightful views surrounded them, but Satya saw little of it. Worries and dangers consumed her thoughts.

They traveled for several hours, stopping to make camp along the sacred river, under a moonlit sky brimming with bright stars. Satya-vatī stepped out of the carriage and stretched. She went down to the river and splashed refreshing, clear water on her face.

The prince approached and invited her to dine with him and the counselor. She graciously accepted, wondering when they would talk about important details.

After a healthy, delicious meal with light conversation, the prince began the serious topics. "Our route will take us through the powerful Pañcāla kingdom that borders the Kurus on our southeast flank."

Satya looked surprised. "The Pañcālas are traditional rivals of the Kurus. Is the best route to travel through their country?"

Bhīṣma nodded. "Yes, it is. After much work, my father recently forged an alliance with the Pañcāla king, Somaka. And now, we must strengthen that alliance by a state visit, if you don't mind."

"Of course not! That is excellent news!" Satya-vatī cried. Pañcāla was an ally of Cedi, loyal to Vasu. She sincerely praised Pañcāla's alliance with the Kurus, but also worried if this would weaken in any way the alliance with Cedi. What did her brothers think? Surely, they knew all about this.

But she said the right things to Deva-vrata. "I congratulate your father on this alliance. The Pañcālas are a key political and military power. I confess that I did not fully appreciate your father's efforts to forge alliances."

The prince smiled. "The king told me about his talks with you, and how your astute arguments influenced him."

"Some of my arguments, perhaps," Satya said with a slight blush. "I did express some views rather imprudently, if not impudently."

The two men laughed and assured her that Śan-tanu thought highly of her perspicacity. "We hope," the counselor said, "that you will not mind the short delay occasioned by our visit to Pañcāla."

"Not at all," Satya said. "I see that policy and protocol require this visit to King Somaka. The age-old rivalry of the Kurus and Pañcālas, alternating between conflict and alliance, is well known. Somaka is a most valuable ally, who must be kept satisfied. So, yes! Let us visit Pañcāla."

The prince and his counselor exchanged smiles of appreciation. The prince thanked her and praised her insight into political affairs.

"On my way here," he added, "on the plea of an urgent affair, I bypassed Pañcāla. I cannot bypass Pañcāla twice without offending its proud ruler and arousing his suspicion. And given the delicate state of the new Kuru-Pañcāla alliance, we must stop."

Satya understood. Deva-vrata had charged down to Kalpi to save his father's heart. He had not thought of international diplomacy. But now he must think of it, or the very father he strove to please would be disturbed by a threat to his new alliance.

"I look forward to our visit," Satya said emphatically, intrigued by this opportunity to participate in strategic diplomacy, following her parents' example. This visit would also furnish her the opportunity to survey Pañcāla's loyalty to Cedi.

But a most delicate concern worried her, and she could not avoid expressing it. "I welcome the Kuru alliance with Pañcāla. But does Śan-tanu know with absolute certainty that King Somaka is devoted to the cause of the Devas?"

"You raise a crucial concern," Śarma said gravely. "Our king is indeed convinced that King Somaka is not an Asura, or a friend of the Asuras. As you know, the Kuru king spent his last life in the Deva world, and he retains his friendship with the Devas. So, with his own superior power of perception, and in consultation with the Devas, he has confirmed that King Somaka is a man to be trusted. Hence, he proceeded with the alliance. Still, your caution and concern do you credit."

Glancing at Śarma, who nodded, the prince said, "Forgive me, but there is one last matter we must discuss."

Satya-vatī urged him to speak. He did. "As you know, our king worked hard to form an alliance with King Somaka of Pañcāla to strengthen our defense against the Asuras. We know King Somaka. He is cautious, even suspicious, by nature, and he will demand to know precisely whom the Kuru king will marry. His disapproval could ruin the alliance. Forgive us for this indelicacy, but my father revealed only that you come from royal blood, but that he was not at liberty to say more. We know that Somaka will insist on knowing precisely who you are, who your family is. He will then calculate all the political and military ramifications of your marriage to Śan-tanu, his new ally. He must know that you are fully determined to oppose the Asura invasion, which, according to my father, you are aware of. One day, your son will be the Kuru king and thus an ally of Somaka's own son. Thus, your identity is crucial to Somaka, his sons, and his kingdom. Dear Satya-vatī, what shall we say to King Somaka, when we see him tomorrow and he inquires about your identity?"

Startled, trying to keep her composure, Satya-vatī silently rebuked herself for not anticipating this inevitable obstacle. Now, she must answer. But what could she say? She would never endanger her son, Vyāsa, by revealing his identity. But if she did not reveal her identity, she might destroy a crucial alliance and thus endanger the world.

The prince and counselor watched and waited. Satya could find no words to speak. Tension mounted in painful silence. She could bring her son this moment and reveal the truth. But no! The Kurus would see as duplicity her long concealment of her son. She would lose their trust.

Yet she must say something. But what? Suddenly, a tiger roared in the night. With blurring speed, twenty Kuru warriors pulled twenty razor-edged swords from their sheaths. Ten of them instantly formed a protective circle around Satya-vatī and the counselor. Ten more ran toward the tiger, their weapons gleaming in the moonlight.

"Excuse me, Your Highness," the prince said to Satya. "The tiger may be an Asura, so I will join my men and take a look."

Deva-vrata's muscles bulged to frightening dimensions as he drew out his sword and followed his men. The tiger gave a defiant roar and fled, his sound trailing, then vanishing into the night.

When the prince returned, Satya-vatī thanked him and his men for protecting her. With a sudden, canny thought, she said, "I'm afraid the tiger unsettled me.

Please, let me retire for the evening and rest. In the morning, before we leave, I will tell you exactly who I am."

Finding this request quite reasonable, and truly concerned for her peace and rest, Deva-vrata and Śarma readily agreed. They had a comfortable tent and bed arranged for her, and urged her not to worry. Formidable Kuru guards would protect her through the night.

Satya-vatī thanked her hosts and explained that she always prayed to Yamunā before sleeping, and she would do that now. The guards kept a respectful distance, as Satya walked to Yamunā's silver, sandy shore. As silver moonlight danced on the river's endless, undulating currents, Satya-vatī, in desperate anxiety, knelt in fervent prayer. All could be lost if she did not reveal her identity, or if she did.

The goddess promised her aid. Satya bowed to Yamunā and sat by her waters, trembling in anxious expectation. She felt a presence by her side. She turned and was startled to see the great sage Parā-śara, father of her child, sitting beside her, just as he did in Kalpi.

CHAPTER 29

Satya gasped, clasped her hands, and bowed to the sage. He bowed in return, and gazed at her with deep concern. "Dear Satya-vatī," he began, "no one but you can see me. But speak softly, lest the guards hear you."

"Of course. Thank you so much for coming."

Parā-śara smiled. "I come with joyous news that will solve the predicament of your identity."

Satya's wide eyes shouted her eagerness to hear the good news. Parā-śara did not keep her waiting. "Satya, our son, Dvaipāyana, has developed his full powers. The Asuras cannot harm him! The world is about to learn that an Avatāra has come!"

Satya made a muffled cry of joy, pressed her hands to her heart and wept. Her son was safe! She gave ardent thanks to Viṣṇu, and to Parā-śara for bringing this ecstatic news. She cried out in a whisper, "Our son is safe! He is safe!"

"Yes, Viṣṇu protected him."

"Yes! And Śan-tanu and his son will protect me. So, I can reveal myself. But how will I explain the past — that my parents concealed my identity? Parā-śara, I still cannot tell the Kurus about our son. I confess that my attachment to Śan-tanu is strong, and the world needs a Kuru-Cedi alliance. Śan-tanu also had a previous union, and child, so he could hardly fault me, especially when I acted within a divine mission. Yet, even if Śan-tanu would accept me, the citizens might not."

"Very true," Parā-śara said. "We know that society is often neither rational nor fair in such matters."

"And we have no time to reform society," Satya said.

"No, we certainly don't."

"It pains me to deceive Śan-tanu, but for a higher cause, I must. And you agree, Parā-śara?"

"I do. There is far too much at stake. Everything is at stake, the three worlds. Future generations will know how you gave birth to an Avatāra, and they will celebrate you. But now is not the time."

"Then how will Bhīṣma and Śarma present me to King Somaka? How will I explain a lifetime incognito?"

Parā-śara smiled. "Satya-vatī, you are brilliant in matters of state. What do you suggest?"

Satya smiled at his compliment. "I will speak the truth, as far as I can. Lord Indra personally chose me to participate in a vital mission to stop the Asuras. He then decreed that for this mission, I must live incognito in my childhood. The Kurus will assume that mission to be a marriage to Śan-tanu. But will they believe me?"

Parā-śara smiled. "Yes, they will. As you said, your words are true, even if others misinterpret them."

With great relief and confidence, and seeing no better solution to a critical situation, Satya thanked Parā-śara from her heart. He thanked her in turn, and said, "I know that you long to see your son, so before I go, I will show you how well he is doing.

They sat by the Yamunā, as they did in Kalpi. Eyes closed, Satya fixed her mind on Parā-śara's words. They carried her high up in the Himālaya, where the Devī of wisdom, Sarasvatī, sends her crystalline river water flowing down to the plains. On the river's western bank, in a grove of jujube trees dotted with bright red fruit, lay a hermitage called Śamyā-prāsa, for it extended as far as a strong man could hurl a staff.

There sat the young Avatāra, Dvaipāyana, facing east over the waters. His long brown locks of hair fell over his shoulders as he meditated on the arduous task of dividing and arranging the Veda. The āśrama bristled with spiritual power.

The vision vanished. Satya-vatī opened her eyes. As tears rolled down her cheeks, she thanked Parā-śara earnestly for the news and vision he brought her.

Choked up with love for her son, Satya-vatī whispered, "When will the world know that an Avatāra has come?"

Parā-śara smiled. "Very soon, I assure you."

"Will he directly oppose the Asuras?"

Parā-śara smiled. "Those like you who know of the Asura invasion will correctly surmise that the Avatāra will help to defend Earth and the three worlds."

With deep apprehension, Satya asked, "Will Dvaipāyana directly fight the Asuras?"

Parā-śara shook his head. "No. Fighting is not a sage's Dharma. And Vyāsa descended to this world to teach Dharma."

Satya-vatī sighed with relief. "Of course. Precisely."

"Our son will prepare the way for Viṣṇu by educating all the good people of Earth. When Viṣṇu comes and acts, Dvaipāyana will then chronicle Viṣṇu's deeds, to guide and inspire the world, and countless future generations." Parā-śara smiled. "Your son will do something else that I hope will please you. He will tell your story, past, present, and future. By his words, you will live in history for thousands of years. All the world will celebrate you."

Amazed, Satya-vatī thanked Parā-śara. But she had one lingering doubt. He urged her to disclose it.

"Parā-śara," she said, "have you told me all that our son will do? Or is there even more to his mission?"

"There is more. Forgive me, Satya, but for now, I cannot reveal it. Just remember your son's promise. When you most need help, call him in your mind, and he will come. I'm sorry I can say no more."

Satya felt a foreboding, as if Parā-śara hinted at future trouble. But she knew that for some higher purpose, he could say no more at this time. She understood, but it made her anxious.

He now begged her leave. With mutual goodwill and affection, and knowing that they must part, the parents of an Avatāra bid each other farewell. Parā-śara vanished as quickly as he had appeared.

Satya-vatī again found herself alone on the riverbank. It was her last evening with dear Yamunā, who had watched over her since birth.

She sat silent on the riverbank, overcome with joy and worry. Above all, her son was safe, beyond the Asura reach. The counter-insurgency, led by her father for many years, had received a most important reinforcement in her son!

But for all her joy, thoughts of the next day worried her. For most of her life, she thought herself a simple, if frustrated, fisher girl. Then she was stunned to learn she was the emperor's daughter, born to play a key role in saving Earth. Out of necessity, she scrupulously kept this secret within her family. But now, the world would learn her real identity. Her life would never be the same.

CHAPTER 30

The next morning, as promised, Satya-vatī revealed to Bhīṣma and Śarma the truth of her identity. She was the only daughter of Emperor Vasu and Empress Girikā. In response to their utter astonishment, she assured them that her five brothers, kings of unquestioned integrity, would happily confirm the fact.

The two men strongly protested the idea that they might doubt her word and require confirmation from others. But they did ask why her identity was so long concealed. Fully prepared, Satya explained that Indra himself had ordered her concealment, knowing that she would play a key role in the counter-insurgency against the Asuras. Indra judged the stratagem necessary, to protect her and the mission. There were further pertinent details that she was not at liberty to disclose.

Prince Bhīṣma shouted, "Of course! It's so clear! Indra chose you to unite the two most powerful dynasties. That's why you had to be concealed, so that you could marry my father. That was the reason. I can see that Providence led me to renounce my throne!"

Sacred duty rendered Satya-vatī powerless to correct the young prince's misinterpretation, which she herself had induced. Behind her gracious, grateful exterior, Satya-vatī grieved terribly. She blamed herself, not Providence, for Bhīṣma's misfortune. It was her blunder to seek her foster parents' blessing for her union with Śan-tanu. She had never ceased rebuking herself for that tragic mistake.

Bhīṣma and Śarma jubilantly bowed to her. They proclaimed the glorious news to the Kuru officers and their men. Joy filled the camp. Soldiers bowed, and gazed at her with awe, wonderstruck to be in the presence of great Vasu's daughter. Satya-vatī sighed. This was but a sample of more celebrity to come.

She recalled with nostalgia her quiet life alone, moving her little boat through Yamunā's waters. That life could never return.

This permanent change in life was then accentuated when Śarma most respectfully informed the princess that the Kurus brought for her, if she would kindly accept their gift, fine garments fit for a princess, and appropriate for a state visit to Pañcāla. Satya-vatī quickly perused the wardrobe and chose a simple yet elegant dress, suitable for a sensible princess, and a minimum of jewelry to avoid being so plain as to draw unwanted curiosity. She dressed quickly, as she always did, thinking deeply about all that had taken place, and all that was about to happen.

Bugles broke through her reverie, signaling imminent departure. Kuru soldiers fell into line with a speed and precision that impressed even a princess. Satya-vatī bid a tearful farewell to dear Yamunā.

With sharp commands and more blasts of bugles and conches, with a strong wind flapping their bright Kuru flags, the party left the river behind. With a lurch, her carriage found the royal road and headed due north toward Kāmpilya, the ancient capital of Pañcāla, standing on the bank of another river, Gaṅgā, whose goddess was Śan-tanu's first wife.

After all the excitement of the last twenty-four hours, it was only now that Satya-vatī remembered with horror what should have been fixed constantly in her mind, from the moment she heard of Prince Deva-vrata's terrible vows. As the carriage rocked and swayed along the road, Satya recalled with a shudder that Śan-tanu explicitly promised to marry her on the condition that she accept Deva-vrata as the future king. Satya-vatī had happily agreed. This was not the first time the thought came to her mind, but now, in the first moment of calm in many hours, she saw with devastating clarity that Śan-tanu had never agreed to marry her under the present conditions, even if arranged by his own son. Deva-vrata had renounced the throne. But in doing so, he had also destroyed the possibility of Satya-vatī complying with Śan-tanu's clear condition.

Other concerns tormented her. The Kuru people would soon hear about all that transpired in the fishing village of Kalpi. Her heart trembled at this. Surely the Kurus, royals and citizens alike, would bitterly resent that Satya's foster father had robbed their beloved prince of his throne, and indeed of a happy life. All for her sake! How could they not loathe her? They would certainly loathe her.

Yet another concern wracked her heart. Considering the apparent fragility of the new Kuru-Pañcāla alliance, Śan-tanu might consider it strategically more desirable to marry a Pañcāla princess. After all, a Pañcāla alliance might endure for several generations. In contrast, a Cedi alliance could hardly outlive Satya-vatī's own generation, since powerful Jarā-sandha, the third generation, would inherit Magadha and with it, great power over her other nephews. Thus, the advantage of a multi-generational alliance with Pañcāla, or another pivotal ally, might convince Śan-tanu to marry elsewhere. He had every right, by Dharma, to consider his vow to Satya-vatī void, no longer binding. And his natural anger at the fisher king's nefarious deed might easily motivate him to seek love and alliance elsewhere.

Satya further depressed herself by vividly imagining how Śan-tanu might react emotionally. Even if he still married her, he might do so now merely as a strategic advantage, to beget a new son and heir to continue the Kuru line.

As her carriage rolled along, she saw little of the scenery. When they stopped at a riverside village to dine beneath an early-risen silver moon, Satya labored to feign interest in her companions' questions. They frequently had to repeat their queries before she heard them.

The prince saw her distress and discreetly inquired into its cause. She insisted she was happy, but he was not fooled. At his gentle insistence, she revealed her mind.

"What will the king say when he hears of your fate? He will blame me. He will despise me! Indeed, I despise myself for all the trouble I have caused you."

The prince earnestly assured her that his father would never act like that. "Our lord never blames the innocent, and clearly you are innocent in this and every matter. Śarma and I have both sworn to it in the message we sent to the king. My father is deeply in love with you. He knows your goodness, and often praises it. Even if a doubt should arise, which I consider impossible, King Śan-tanu will believe me and Śarma. I told my father of your concerns, and urged him to send back his approval. I told him our route, and the return messenger will find us as quickly as possible."

Satya-vatī nodded, but then raised the other problem. Even if his father truly accepted her, the citizens, who so loved the prince, must blame and detest her. Here, too, the prince implored her to give up her fears. Kuru citizens would not blame her. "If needed, which is most unlikely, I will make them see the truth. They are fair-minded, like their king. When they see you, and hear you, and learn what actually happened, I know they will love you as I do."

"How can you love me, after what happened? I do not deserve your love. If only there was a way for you to take back your vow. You don't know what you're doing. You're so young. You don't know how you will suffer later in life. Surely, your father did not authorize you to do this."

"No, he did not. But please do not be angry with me. Please accept me as your son, for you shall be my mother. I know you disapprove of my actions. But I beg you, do not reject my father because of what I did."

He then pleaded that if Satya did not come, Deva-vrata would have only added to his father's misery. The king had lost his chosen heir, irrevocably. If Śan-tanu also lost the woman he loved, his misery would be doubled. To obtain an heir, the king might be forced into a loveless marriage.

She could not refute his words. In her mind, she added to them the very real danger to Earth if she failed to unite Kurus and Cedis.

In deep anxiety, she made her decision. She would continue toward Hastinā-pura, but she would not enter the city until she received Śan-tanu's decision. Satya said to the prince, "You must send a message to your father."

"I already did that yesterday."

"Hear me," she replied. "You must send another message, stating clearly that I will travel to the gates of the capital, but I will enter Hastinā-pura only if two conditions are explicitly met. First, I must receive a clear confirmation that the Kuru king will accept my hand in marriage, despite the awful behavior of my foster father, and the grievous injury done to you, which I deeply lament, and for which I am profoundly ashamed."

"I will repeat your words," said the prince, who realized the futility of arguing with the princess.

"And second," she added, "King Śan-tanu and his citizens must accept me without a trace of anger or resentment. If they do in fact resent the great evil of my foster father, I will perfectly understand. I will then humbly beg the Kuru monarch to accept my brothers, the Cedi rulers, as his brothers in arms. I will fall at his feet and beseech him to do this for the good of the world, indeed, of the three worlds. I will then make sure that Śan-tanu is never again troubled by the sight of me, that I never again remind him of the evil I indirectly caused to his beloved son." In fact, Satya-vatī was firmly resolved that if Śan-tanu rejected her, she would flee to a distant land, and place her soul and fate in Viṣṇu's hands.

Bhīṣma strenuously protested her fearful prognosis and drastic contingency plan. "There is no need for such words. Indeed, I cannot send such a message. I'm sure my father will gladly accept you."

Satya insisted with even greater vehemence. "Forgive me, but I shall not enter the Kuru capital until I have received clear assurances that the Kuru king willingly, indeed, gladly accepts both my points. I'm sorry, but I shall not yield on this issue."

"As you wish," Bhīṣma replied. "As you ordered, I shall send your message at once. I will clearly explain our route so that my father's reply may reach us long before we reach the gates of our capital."

They resumed their journey. With all her worries, it was the gates of Kāmpilya that soon commanded Satya's attention. Passing through a Pañcāla forest, she saw Kāmpilya's spires and domes from miles away. This was the ancient capital of a dynasty mentioned even in the Veda. As they came closer, the spires and domes grew to majestic proportions. They passed groves of finely cultivated fruit trees, and entered a broad, shaded avenue that led straight to a majestic city gate, passing under which, one entered the city.

As they approached the city, and the river, whose waters flowed down from Hastinā-pura, Satya glanced at Deva-vrata, who rode beside her on a noble steed. As he approached his mother's river, he bowed, placed his hand over his heart, and kept riding.

A few hundred yards from the city gates, thrilling sounds of a military band greeted them. With its royal colors shining in the sun, the band marched out of the city gates to greet the Kuru party. The royal reception swelled with marching infantry, and expert cavalry on fine horses.

Pañcāla and Kuru flags, ceremonially crossed, tossed about in the breeze. Royal priests rode out on chariots, blessing the visitors with Vedic mantras. For the first time in her life, Satya-vatī was appearing publicly as royalty, as a very respectable member of society.

The king's son and heir, Pṛṣata, greeted his guests at the entrance to the royal palace. The prince deeply admired Bhīṣma, whom he knew by reputation, and whose radiance and stature evinced his demigod origin.

He led them to opulent quarters, according to their rank, where they would bathe and rest after their journey. A large and sumptuous variety of food would be brought to them at their wish.

That evening, the king would personally greet and host them at a state banquet. Prince Deva-vrata, increasingly famous as Bhīṣma, would then formally introduce Princess Satya-vatī to the king, and thereby to the world.

Satya could not suppress her anxiety. For the first time, the world would know her true identity. A single state dinner in Pañcāla would change everything, both in her own life, and potentially in the balance of world power. A king or prince who married Satya-vatī would be intimately connected to the still mighty Cedi dynasty.

As she tried unsuccessfully to rest, awaiting the formal dinner with the king, Satya-vatī realized more than ever that a Kuru-Pañcāla alliance made a Kuru-Cedi alliance even more urgent. Otherwise, the Cedi dynasty might be increasingly marginalized on the world stage.

She was eager to tell her brothers about her apparent marriage to Śan-tanu. They would all come to the wedding. But she must delay her ecstasy and theirs until she knew that Śan-tanu would accept her under these dramatically changed conditions. Her hope and confidence collapsed. She had no final confirmation that Śan-tanu would accept her. How would he react to his son's tragic abdication of the Kuru throne? How would the Kuru nation react? Yet she would very soon be presented to the powerful Pañcāla king as Śan-tanu's bride-to-be. If Śan-tanu rejected her, she would hide from the world for a very long time.

CHAPTER 31

As the senior Kurus entered the banquet hall, a musical ensemble played strings and horns, filling the hall with exquisite melodies and harmonies. Deva-vrata took the seat of honor to the right of the king at a grand table. By the prince's pre-banquet diplomacy, Satya-vatī sat to his right. To the king's left sat his son Pṛṣata, who was a few years older than Deva-vrata. To Pṛṣata's left sat the famous sage Bharad-vāja, his tutor.

As Satya watched the prince interact with his sage tutor, their friendship seemed a model of mutual regard between social classes — a brāhmaṇa and a prince.

The music quieted. King Somaka rose to welcome his guests. He spoke well, in the expected way, praising the Kurus, rejoicing in their alliance, and welcoming King Śan-tanu's bride-to-be. With a telling look at Satya-vatī, he added pointedly that no one in Pañcāla had yet the pleasure of knowing this lovely and fortunate princess. It was Deva-vrata's turn to speak. He had arranged with Satya-vatī that this would be the moment to reveal her identity to the world.

The Kuru prince spoke with consummate skill, strictly following the norms of diplomacy. He first praised King Somaka, recounting his chivalrous deeds and noble character. He then expressed moving gratitude to the Pañcālas for their recent alliance with the Kurus.

Having so far pleased his hosts, Deva-vrata knew that they fully expected a coherent, convincing explanation of two things: first, his abdication as heir apparent to the Kuru throne, and, second, a clear, satisfying identification of the future Kuru queen, a lady whose sons would inherit Kuru power and thus heavily impact Pañcāla.

Bhīṣma began, "The world is quickly learning that I, son of Śan-tanu and Devī Gaṅgā, have renounced the Kuru throne. I did this to ensure my father's marriage to a princess who can have no equal in this world, based on her ability, her beauty, and her lineage."

At these words, King Somaka, his son Pṛṣata, sage Bharad-vāja, and all the Pañcāla nobility, glanced at each other, surprised by this unexpected declaration. They had of course discussed the coming of Śan-tanu's new bride. They had received reports that she was bright and beautiful, but entirely unknown. Thus, they concluded, she was very likely of common birth.

They had decided, in pursuit of vital political interests, to overlook the young lady's non-royal status. They were prepared to be generous and liberal. But Deva-vrata's bold claim that the lady had no equal in lineage startled them, and they knew not how to take it. Perhaps in the throes of his own great loss, Deva-vrata, or Bhīṣma, as he was now apparently called, had lost his reason. Everyone in the Pañcāla contingent knew well the world's leading princesses, and even those of second and third rank. Satya-vatī was unknown, unranked.

Deva-vrata detected, and smiled at, the covert Pañcāla reaction to his words, and he did not keep them in suspense. "I have made," he said calmly, "regarding the lineage of my father's bride, what many might well consider to be a highly exaggerated claim. But I speak the truth, as you will now see."

Deva-vrata paused but for a moment, as his hosts leaned forward in expectation. "King Somaka, surely you agree that the greatest ruler of your father's generation was a man accepted by all as king of kings — glorious Vasu of Cedi."

Here Deva-vrata paused, as Somaka and all his retinue bowed their heads in honor of the departed Vasu.

The Kuru prince continued. "You know — indeed, all the world knows — that great Indra personally established Vasu as emperor of our planet. The world also knows that Vasu and his queen, Girikā, begot five powerful sons, who each rule a kingdom, and who jointly rule their homeland of Cedi. The world knows as well that Vasu and Girikā inspired us all with their ideal example of retiring to the Final Forest in their last years, and devoting themselves to self-realization."

At all these points, the Pañcālas nodded in agreement. After a short pause, Deva-vrata said emphatically, "However, the world does not know that King Vasu and Queen Girikā, during their reign, begot a beautiful daughter, equal to her brothers in character, intelligence, and goodness."

The gathered royalty, ministers, and sages had expected a surprise from Deva-vrata. But none were prepared for a revelation of this magnitude. Shocked into silence, their eyes darted from Deva-vrata, to Satya-vatī, and back to the prince, as they waited, breathless, for more.

With perfect timing, Deva-vrata declared, "Distinguished hosts, your surprise can hardly exceed my own when I first heard this news. But Lord Indra himself ordered that this princess of the first rank be carefully hidden from the world. Why? Because Indra, and perhaps Viṣṇu himself, selected this young lady for a special mission on Earth, a task crucial to our joint defense of this planet. And in the superior judgment of those whom we revere, this mission required that her identity be concealed from the world until today. The reasons for such concealment are known to Indra, who ordered it. We who serve the Devas must assume that his reasons were fully rational."

Deva-vrata had the full attention of his audience. They listened to every word with the focused attention of great yogīs.

"What earthly princess," Bhīṣma declared, "could be more worthy of our respect than great Vasu's daughter, chosen to help save Earth?"

After a brief pause in which he fixed his guests in his riveting gaze, Deva-vrata continued, striking the air with his fist to emphasize his words. "That most exalted princess sits in this hall, at this table, in the sight of all, directly at my side."

Here Bhīṣma turned, and bowed to Satya-vatī. "O worthy king, I have the great honor of presenting to you, to all your court, and to your venerable teachers, the daughter of Vasu and Girikā, Princess Satya-vatī!"

Hardly breathing, King Somaka, his son Pṛṣata, sage Bharad-vāja, and indeed all the Pañcālas present, stared in wide-eyed amazement. Stunning as this revelation was, they could not doubt the words of Gaṅgā's son. Keenly conscious of the need for perfect etiquette, they quickly put aside any trace of incredulity, and bowed with earnest alacrity. The king rose to his feet, and gave high praise to Satya-vatī's parents. He then showered her with respectful kindness.

Perhaps most astonished was Satya-vatī herself. Her astounding metamorphosis from the naive daughter of fishing folk into a most exalted princess, soon to be Kuru Queen, amazed no one more than it amazed Satya-vatī.

After all these formalities, King Somaka announced that Pañcāla would provide entertainment for its honored guests. After the banquet items were expeditiously removed by smartly uniformed attendants, a brilliant show of song, dance, and comedy ensued, ending before the audience could weary of it.

King Somaka, with impeccable decorum, bid his guests goodnight and retired with his queen to their chambers, leaving the two princes to become better acquainted. Serious talks on political and military issues were reserved for the next day.

Satya-vatī remained in the large hall to become better acquainted with some of the leading ladies of Pañcāla, and to discreetly observe the princes. Bhīṣma, who remained extremely influential among the Kurus, though no longer heir apparent, engaged in friendly, animated conversation with Prince Pṛṣata. Both understood the gravity of their alliance, and both did their duty well. A real mutual liking made it all easy.

As she lay down to rest that night in a regal bedroom reserved for high royalty, her worried mind could not rest. One thought would not leave her. Because she was honored now by world leaders as the daughter of Vasu and the betrothed of Śan-tanu, her celebrity would quickly spread to all the kings of the world. She must get word to her brothers.

The next day, in the refreshingly cool air of early morning, Satya walked through the extensive palace gardens. She met Deva-vrata by a fountain, and at her invitation they sat together to speak.

She explained the absolute necessity of informing her brothers about her marriage to Śan-tanu. The prince understood at once, and summoned Kuru envoys in whose intelligence and discretion he fully confided. Satya then dictated a clear message to her brothers.

To ensure their confidence in the authenticity of the message, she included some personal words and anecdotes that only she and her brothers could possibly know. In any case, no one could doubt the veracity of an official Kuru envoy. She sent a few special words to her twin brother, Matsya, whom she especially missed. The envoys would leave within the hour.

After this, Satya-vatī and Deva-vrata sat for a breakfast of more varieties of fruit than Satya-vatī thought possible on one planet, along with milk, yogurt, nuts, breads, hot cereals, and varieties of sweets. An hour later, the Pañcāla royalty, with top ministers and advisers, met with Deva-vrata, Satya-vatī, and Śarma.

Everyone in the room saw the importance of a union between the Kuru king and the late emperor's daughter, especially given the new Kuru-Pañcāla alliance. Asuras would have to delay their aggression. Pious rulers would be thrilled and emboldened. Everyone would have to adapt to the new political-military reality.

Should Satya-vatī's marriage to Śan-tanu take place, the kings of the world would journey to Hastinā-pura for the most momentous wedding of their generation, a union that would redefine global power. However, the Pañcālas did not suspect, as Satya-vatī did, that Śan-tanu might not react well to the heartbreaking injustice done to his son.

In that meeting of leaders, only Satya-vatī worried that although Śan-tanu was a good man, an excellent man, he was also a proud, fierce warrior and king. His personal choice of an heir had been sabotaged by the machinations of a crude fisherman. Satya-vatī remembered the violent pride she detected in Śan-tanu, despite his efforts to control and conceal it, when the fisher king affronted him and demanded impossible conditions.

But now was not the time or place for Satya-vatī to raise those issues. She did participate in the general discussions, often making intelligent, well-considered points.

As the meeting ended, King Somaka affectionately smiled at her and said, "Dear girl, your father was always most kind to me and my father. He protected us like his own family. You will always be most welcome here, Satya-vatī, as an honored and cherished guest. Indeed, your exalted father has come to us through you. Having met you, I have no doubt that this extraordinary union by marriage of the Kuru and Cedi dynasties will establish a strong bond between all three of our realms. For Pañcāla, to have King Vasu present in our alliance, through his daughter, is a real blessing. It gives us confidence."

With real affection and respect, Satya-vatī thanked King Somaka for his kind words about her father. She vowed with everything in her power to continue her father's good work in the world. Bhīṣma and Śarma carefully observed this dialogue, and were highly impressed with Satya-vatī's expertise and contribution to crucial international affairs.

Somaka looked at the Kuru prince and his advisor and pointedly said, "Vasu was king of kings, yet he was always kind to us. He never used his power to dominate his friends. He never interfered in their kingdoms. Only when a ruler mistreated his citizens, or sought to oppress other kingdoms — only then did Vasu intervene. He saw himself as a servant of every king who served the Law, Dharma. Like a kindly father, he ruled for our good, without personal ambition."

Satya-vatī understood that by sincerely praising her father, Somaka made clear the terms under which he would continue as a faithful ally of the Cedis and Kurus. Deva-vrata then expressed his full support for Satya-vatī's words, and Vasu's policies, making clear to Somaka that the Kurus would indeed follow Vasu's method.

Deva-vrata said, "King Somaka, I eagerly came to your great kingdom precisely to give you and your government every assurance of my father's full dedication to his friendship and alliance with you and your realm. We honor and emulate the spirit of King Vasu."

The Pañcāla king smiled, and glanced at Satya-vatī, as if inviting her to speak. She did so at once. "Somaka Mahārāja, kindly permit me to speak on behalf of my brothers, heirs to my father, Vasu."

"You would honor us by doing so," the king said.

Satya-vatī then reassured him that all her brothers spoke highly of Pañcāla and especially of its king. "The Cedis are bound by honor, interest, and sincere friendship to the Pañcālas. Further, the Cedis are most eager to strengthen that friendship."

"Before we end this encouraging meeting," Somaka said, "I will speak to you on a topic that directly and dramatically affects all of us. An Avatāra has come to our world."

The news stunned Bhīṣma and Śarma, and all the Pañcāla leaders present. Satya easily expressed surprise, since she was truly surprised that the news had spread so quickly. Sly Parā-śara had told her just the day before that the world would learn of the Avatāra very soon.

Bhīṣma said to the king, "Are you absolutely sure?"

Somaka nodded. "Yes, I am. In Pañcāla, we pride ourselves on the quality and efficiency of our intelligence-gathering. The information I gave you is reliable and accurate. I'm sure your father, King Śan-tanu, has just received the same information, and will very soon disclose it to you. Indeed, the news is spreading like fire."

"Who is the Avatāra, and what will he do in this world?" Śarma asked.

The Pañcāla prince's tutor, sage Bharad-vāja, replied. "We all know that for generations, fewer and fewer people, even many brāhmaṇas, fully understand the Veda, even though it has guided our civilization since time began. We understand Law from the Veda. If we lose our grasp of the Law, we will surely violate it, or fail to act upon it. Civilization will grow weak and confused. We will be prey for the Asuras."

Bharad-vāja looked around the room. Everyone nodded their grave assent. The sage went on. "In every cycle of ages, an Avatāra comes to divide, arrange, and explain the Veda. That Avatāra is called Vyāsa, 'the Arranger.' Asura threat makes it urgent that people return to the Law. For the Law, Dharma, preserves those who preserve it. The Law surely breaks those who break it."

The Pañcālas and Kurus glanced gravely at each other, and at Satya-vatī.

"I understand," said Somaka. "I really do. My priests barely grasp the Veda. They have, of course, mastered the rites and mantras. And they extract from them worldly power. But the moral essence — the higher vision of the soul, and its power — that is fading. Without true spiritual power, we cannot defeat the Asuras. The Avatāra has come at the right time, no doubt. His title is Vyāsa. But what is his name?"

Bharad-vāja replied. "His personal name is said to be Dvaipāyana, for he was born on an island, a dvīpa."

Satya-vatī shook inside, but fought to preserve a calm exterior.

"But where? Which island?" Bhīṣma asked.

Satya feigned a lively curiosity as her heart raced.

"No one knows," Prince Pṛṣata said.

Satya-vatī breathed a sigh of relief.

"Who are the Avatāra's parents?" Counselor Śarma asked. Satya feared he looked straight at her as he spoke these words. Did he know about her divine child? Would he reveal it to everyone?

Satya-vatī, hardly breathing, looked so pale that Prince Bhīṣma leaned over and whispered to her, "Are you all right? You look ill."

"I'm very well," she gasped. "Just a little tired from the journey."

"Now that is the strangest thing," King Somaka said, not noticing Satya-vatī. "The sages claim that the Avatāra's father is the legendary Parā-śara. But no one has any idea who his mother is. That is the real mystery. Parā-śara left this planet without telling anyone. How could such an exalted woman remain unknown? It's hard to fathom. Don't you agree, Princess?"

"It is hard indeed," she said, trying to speak in a normal voice.

"The sages do agree on one point," the king said. "The Avatāra is so powerful, though still young, that the Asuras will not challenge him. Oh, and they also say that Vyāsa, or Dvaipāyana, will do other things to defeat the Asuras. But no one knows any details. That is another mystery."

After everyone gave thanks to Viṣṇu for the appearance of an Avatāra, the meeting ended in high spirits and mutual cordiality. The state visit to Kāmpilya, now ending, was a grand success.

The Kurus planned to leave after lunch. King Somaka wanted his guests to see his northern capital, Ahi-cchatra. It was the Pañcāla city closest to Hastinā-pura and therefore a key link in the alliance. Prince Pṛṣata and his friend Bharad-vāja would accompany the Kurus there personally to see to their reception and accommodations, and show them the city that was a strategic component of the Pañcāla-Kuru alliance.

As she prepared to leave Kāmpilya, Satya-vatī compared it in her mind to the Cedi capital of Śukti-matī. The two cities were of similar size and opulence. Satya noted with increased respect for her parents that they had not exploited their imperial position to accrue personal wealth, or to unnecessarily control others, or even to embellish their capital beyond other capitals. As king of kings, Vasu served others, and acted in everyone's interest.

With fine ceremony, and sincere words, Somaka bid farewell to the Kurus and Satya-vatī. His son, Prince Pṛṣata, and a royal entourage escorted his guests to Ahi-cchatra, which was smaller than the capital, but equally attractive. Still, it could not dazzle an emperor's daughter. Satya took care to say all the right things and fully pleased her hosts.

Pṛṣata settled his guests in beautiful lodgings, personally showed them the city, and held a banquet in their honor. The next morning, after sincere exchanges of gifts, thanks, and invitations, the Kurus set off for Hastinā-pura, the grandest of all cities. Despite her worries, Satya felt a thrill as the Kuru Prince thundered a command, and the whole party set out with all the pomp and splendor of ancient Kuru tradition.

But the thrill soon vanished. Satya-vatī's anxiety steadily increased as they journeyed toward the Kuru capital. No reply had come from Śan-tanu.

Satya-vatī had made it clear that she would not enter the city of Hastinā-pura without the full assurances she had requested. She must receive Śan-tanu's heartfelt acceptance of her as his bride. A rejection from Śan-tanu would send her fleeing back to a lonely, loveless life in the forest. But it would be a life with dignity. She still believed in Parā-śara's promise of a happy and strategic marriage, and, if necessary, she would await that boon in sad but principled seclusion.

But Śan-tanu's rejection would discourage other respectable monarchs from seeking her hand. They would fear offending or displeasing the Kuru king, or embarrassing themselves by accepting a woman that a more respected monarch rejected. They might also assume that wise Śan-tanu surely had excellent reasons to reject her.

Were Śan-tanu to reject her, that might even taint the Cedi dynasty. Kings might feel that they must choose between the Kurus and the Cedis, and at this point in history, most might choose the Kurus. This would weaken the Cedi dynasty and leave it vulnerable to a hundred misfortunes.

Satya-vatī shook her head, as if to shake out these dark thoughts. She thought instead of Viṣṇu, his goodness and power. Cedi power was born in service to Viṣṇu, as mediated by Indra. If Cedi was to continue, at least in this generation, to be a major force for good in the world, they only needed Viṣṇu's support. Her father, Vasu, had done so much to protect Viṣṇu's brāhmaṇas. Viṣṇu would not forget that devoted service.

By now, Śan-tanu must know everything. Soon, she would know his decision. He must accept her, or another wife, to secure a Kuru heir. Bhīṣma would not go back on his word.

Satya-vatī yearned to believe Bhīṣma's assurances that his father would love her as before. He must know his own father. But how could the Kuru king, however noble, love her as before, after the evil done by her foster father? And if Śan-tanu married her just to produce an heir, that would break her heart. Parā-śara had promised she would find love, and love must be reciprocal, or it is constant hurt.

Suddenly, in the distance, the pounding rhythm of hooves, and swirling clouds of dust drove away all other thoughts. Kuru guards sprang into formation, with Bhīṣma at their head. Satya strained her eyes till their object came clearly into focus. A disciplined cavalry unit, boasting bright Kuru colors, approached at a gallop. Streaming over the horizon, blasting the air with bugles and conches, they rode straight toward Satya's contingent.

Deva-vrata smiled broadly and gave a thundering blast with his own conch. Satya's heart beat fast as the riders raced toward them. Surely they brought news from Hastinā-pura. From Śan-tanu!

Satya's fate, and perhaps that of the world, rested in messages soon to be revealed by fast-riding Kuru envoys. She must remain calm. She must not disgrace her family by letting the Kurus see an emperor's daughter in such an agitated state. Her thoughts flew to her noble parents, to her brothers, especially Matsya, and finally to Viṣṇu, her shelter of last resort.

ACKNOWLEDGMENTS

I offer my heartfelt thanks to many persons whose valuable help made this publication possible. This list includes Bob Cohen (Brahma Tirtha) who has rendered a lifetime of valuable assistance to all my projects; Sol Maria Videla (Pancali Devi) who brilliantly manages all of my global publications; Tal Patalon (Taruni Devi) who rendered valuable help in many ways—organizational, inspirational, and financial—with both the print and audio books; Natacha Bourgel (Naṭeśa Devi) who expertly and devotedly dealt with all the legal affairs of this and other publications, as well as helping in getting the book ready for print. I am always grateful to Śyāmala Kiśorī for her insightful comments on this book and my other books; Sivan Gazit and Shivanand Sharma who offered many valuable suggestions; Adriana Landívar (Adri-līlā Devī) for her excellent, enthusiastic production of all the historical maps in this volume; and Susan Shapiro (Surabhi) who generously helped with the editing. I also offer my sincere thanks to many others whose names are not mentioned here. I am truly blessed to be in such good, expert, and generous company.

READ MORE FROM HOWARD RESNICK, A. K. A. H. D. GOSWAMI

Justin Davis (English. Spanish and Portuguese translations available)

A Comprehensive Guide to Bhagavad-gītā with Literal Translation (English. Spanish, Portuguese, German, Italian, French, Hebrew, and Turkish translations available)

Quest for Justice: Select Tales with Modern Illuminations from the Mahabharata (English. Spanish and Portuguese translations available)

Enlightenment by the Natural Path (English. Spanish translation available)

Episodios do Mahabharata (Portuguese)

Vida (Portuguese. Spanish translation also available)

A Meta Da Vida: Questionamentos sobre o que Realmente Somos (Portuguese. Spanish translation available)

Os Valores da Liberdade: Onde o Ocidente Encontra o Oriente (Portuguese. Spanish translation available)

Placer Infinito Verdad Absoluta (Portuguese. Spanish translation available)

Razão & Divindade (Portuguese. Spanish translation available)

Soluçoes (3 volumes)

Srimad Bhagavatam — Tenth Canto (English)

Srimad Bhagavatam — Eleventh Canto (English)

Srimad Bhagavatam — Twelfth Canto (English)

Readers interested in the subject matter of this book or wishing to correspond with the author are invited to write to bookinfo@hdgoswami.com.

MANDALA
An Imprint of MandalaEarth
PO Box 3088
San Rafael, CA 94912
www.MandalaEarth.com

Find us on Facebook: www.facebook.com/MandalaEarth

Publisher Raoul Goff
Associate Publisher Phillip Jones
Editorial Director Katie Killebrew
Editorial Assistant Amanda Nelson
VP, Creative Director Chrissy Kwasnik
Art Director Ashley Quackenbush
Senior Designer Stephanie Odeh
VP Manufacturing Alix Nicholaeff
Production Manager Joshua Smith
Sr Production Manager, Subsidiary Rights Lina s Palma-Temena

Cover illustration by Onkar Fondekar

HDG GLOBAL PUBLICATIONS

Published in partnership with HDG Global Publications

ISBN: 979-8-88762-073-2
ISBN: 979-8-88762-150-0 (Export Edition)

Manufactured in India by Insight Editions
10 9 8 7 6 5 4 3 2 1

ROOTS of PEACE REPLANTED PAPER

Mandala Publishing, in association with Roots of Peace, will plant two trees for each tree used in the manufacturing of this book. Roots of Peace is an internationally renowned humanitarian organization dedicated to eradicating land mines worldwide and converting war-torn lands into productive farms and wildlife habitats. Roots of Peace will plant two million fruit and nut trees in Afghanistan and provide farmers there with the skills and support necessary for sustainable land use.

FSC
www.fsc.org
MIX
Paper | Supporting responsible forestry
FSC® C016779